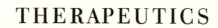

THERAPEUTICS

THERAPEUTICS

FROM THE PRIMITIVES TO THE 20TH CENTURY

WITH AN APPENDIX: HISTORY OF DIETETICS

Erwin H. Ackerknecht, M.D.

Hafner Press
A DIVISION OF MACMILLAN PUBLISHING CO., INC.
New York

COLLIER MACMILLAN PUBLISHERS
London

Translated from the original German edition: "Erwin H. Ackernecht. Therapie von den Primitiven bis zum 20. Jahrhundert" published in 1970 by Ferdinand Enke Verlag, Stuttgart, Germany.

HAFNER PRESS
A Division of Macmillan Publishing Co., Inc.
866 Third Avenue, New York, N.Y. 10022.
Collier-Macmillan Canada, Ltd., Toronto, Ontario

Library of Congress Catalog Card Number: 72–88252
ISBN: 02–840060–7

Printed in the United States of America

In Memory of GEORGE URDANG
Tilsit 1882 — Madison, Wis. 1960

Contents

Preface

FOR MANY years I have felt that a history of therapeutics would be the most useful book a medical historian could write. Therapeutics still is something that can be only very partially learned from books or lectures. Under the pressure of the patients' suffering and influenced by many suggestions in periodicals and advertising, the young physician generally develops a somewhat hectic activity which is not always as useful as he intends, and which, after several decades of experience, he changes rather thoroughly.

I have written this book in the hope that a study of our collective experience will save for at least some young physicians and their patients some years of unnecessary personal experience. To write such a book seemed all the more justified as, since Julius Petersen's *Hauptmomente in der geschichtlichen Entwicklung der medizinischen Therapie* (Copenhagen, 1877), no such book has appeared. For many years I have collected materials for this book, and I intended to write it in the form of my books on Virchow and the "Parisian Medicine." My state of health makes this impossible. I have therefore decided to publish my materials in a shorter form with only a selective bibliography, and I do hope that this shorter book will nevertheless be of service.

In this history of therapeutics, I must assume a certain rudimentary knowledge of the general history of medicine, especially of theories and discoveries. Several short books exist in which these data can be found. I had to avoid padding this book with these data if it was to serve its purpose. It was furthermore impossible to make this a history of all therapeutic methods. To these belongs surgery, and a discussion of surgery would transgress the limits of this book and my own competence. Essentially this is a history of therapeutics in internal diseases, especially pharmacotherapy. I have nevertheless briefly mentioned the status of surgery, psychotherapeutics, and other therapeutic methods, as I did not want the reader to forget that therapeutics is more than only pharmacotherapy.

Several years ago I suggested that we medical historians should be more concerned with what actually happened to the patient than with studying exclusively medical classics. I feel guilty of not always having followed my own prescription.

Due to lack of space, quacks and secret remedies have not been discussed in more detail, although, at certain times and at certain places, they were undoubtedly and still are major elements of therapeutics. Unscientific behavior has apparently at all times and by many patients of all social strata been regarded as psychologically particularly satisfactory. Quackish behavior can very well be combined with the possession of an M.D. diploma.

I am, of course, not unaware of the fact that therapeutics with its increasing efficiency has sometimes become a problem in itself. Is the treatment of many incurables and disabled always meaningful and humane? This is not a historic problem, and I do not believe that it is the task of doctors to decide this matter anyhow. The doctor is no judge, and he owes to the patient all available therapeutics.

In spite of these limitations, I hope that the book will fulfill its purpose. Dietetics has played such an important role in therapeutics that it seemed to me desirable to discuss its history separately in an appendix.

I would like to thank my colleague, Professor Dr. H. M. Koelbing, and my wife, Edith, for criticism of the manuscript and many suggestions. Likewise I am grateful to my collaborators, Dr. Esther Fischer-Homberger and Dr. Alfred W. Gubser.

Introduction

MEN HAVE been persecuted and tormented by disease since their beginning on earth. In their fight against disease they guessed or invented and transmitted therapeutics. From the point of view of society as well as of the individual patient, therapeutics and prevention are undoubtedly the most important aspects of medicine. But medical history has dealt with both only sparingly.

Some of the reasons therefore are obvious in the case of therapeutics. Even if one does not want to go as far as the Bonn clinician Martini, who calls the history of therapeutics a history of errors, it must be admitted that, till recently, therapeutics was undoubtedly the weakest point of medicine. Diagnostics and physiology were long before far better developed. And nobody likes to talk of one's weak points. But the situation has changed so much during the past decades that some have already spoken of our period as the epoch of therapeutics. Causal treatment has now replaced in many cases symptomatic treatment which, for millennia, was the main focus of therapeutics. Thereby one of the difficulties in writing a history of therapeutics has disappeared.

Aside from its problematic results achieved in the past, there is another reason why historians dislike dealing with the history of therapeutics. The history of therapeutics is embarrassing on account of the extraordinary lack of logic, rationality, and openness to experience that is manifest in its course. This should perhaps have been just the reason to study the history of therapeutics more thoroughly! These studies could perhaps have contributed more to the practical education of young physicians than the history of any other aspect of medicine.

Insofar as therapeutics depends on technological and scientific

1

progress, methods have improved tremendously during the last centuries, and the problems changed continuously. The same holds for the economic aspects. In as much as therapeutics depends on human judgment—and it does, of course, to a large extent—the problems remain the same, and the same human insufficiencies have the tendency to produce the same regrettable results over and over again. In this context I will never forget an episode twenty years ago in the United States which took place after one of the early and obviously overenthusiastic reports on the results of cortisone. Several of my colleagues approached me and said quite seriously and melancholically: "Well, Erwin, you will probably soon be the only man left on this faculty." I could reassure them. But it is almost unbelievable that these experienced men could believe in all earnestness that cortisone could solve all medical problems in the near future.

As therapeutics is supposedly based on experience, the study of its history is a valuable contribution to the knowledge of the nature of human experience in general. The history of therapeutics also reflects all too clearly the human inclination to act according to fashion.

It seems to be a regrettable historical "law" that the bad is not at all caused only by those who intend to do so, but that, quite the contrary, the bad arises very often from erroneous attempts to do the good. Unfortunately the history of therapeutics gives numerous examples for this "law."

How are we to explain the many reports of success contained in the history of therapeutics where quite obviously the therapeutics applied could not have produced this success? It seems to me that four main reasons exist for these reports: (1) A wrong diagnosis. If "cancer" was not cancer, it could easily be cured by carrot juice. (2) Spontaneous recovery, which is possible in all diseases. (3) The curative effect of suggestion, which exists in psychical as well as in physical disease and which seems all the stronger if patient and doctor are not conscious of this fact. (4) The forgetting of failures or the reinterpretation of such.

The regrettable facts of the history of therapeutics illustrate indirectly the great tenacity of the human organism. If we have to report critically the actions of many therapists of the past, we should try to avoid any kind of self-righteousness. Faced by the sick, the doctor is under enormous pressure to do "something," and this "something" can be very easily in error.

It is often very difficult to decide what the relationship is between theories that accompany therapeutics and practice itself. Are these theories actually decisive for the applied treatment, are they the "ratio," or are they only rationalizations to justify the use of methods and materials that are much older than the theory? Temkin has shown this very well in the case of the use of cathartics and antiepileptic drugs before and after Galen. Whether ratio or rationalization, these theories announce in any case the existence of certain therapeutic practices and serve therefore in the reconstruction of the therapeutic past. But in such a reconstruction we have to be careful not to overlook such therapeutic measures as were applied and are applied without any theory.

It is obvious that therapeutic opportunities have changed tremendously during the past decades. Therefore the attitude of physicians today can no longer be as skeptical or reserved, as might very often have been the correct position in the past. We therefore cannot advocate the same attitudes in the present, although even today the Hippocratic rule to "be useful or at least do no harm" should be binding for any physician.

I

Primitive Therapeutics

THE ONLY existing clear evidence of therapeutics of early men at our disposal is the trephined skulls of the Neolithic. But a study of the therapeutics of "savages" or "primitives," reported abundantly by ethnologists and missionaries during the past two hundred years, allows us to gain an approximate notion of the therapeutics of early men. Both groups, early men and primitives, lived on about the same technological and ideological level.

We begin by enumerating the almost exclusively symptomatic therapeutic methods of primitives. They have numerous drugs which are taken as powders, pills, infusions, decoctions, fumigations, cataplasms, inhalations, and clysters, i.e., in the same forms that are still used today. They lack only injections, of which they are afraid because they suspect the simultaneous injection of a disease demon. Among the drugs to be discussed here in detail we find numerous cathartics, emetics, antispasmodics, cough mixtures, and diuretics. i.e., drugs that "clean" the body materially and ritually. Primitives maintain diets and use massage, baths, sweats, cupping, sucking, scarification, and bleeding. They have a very rudimentary surgery, which is above all wound treatment. Some have incubators out of fear of the ghosts of the premature child. Some run away in the case of infectious disease; others isolate or even vaccinate against such and against snakebite. Seen from our point of view they practice above all psychotherapy by means of suggestion and confession, often in the form of group treatment.

At the same time these therapeutics contain numerous magicoreligious elements, like music with drums and rattles, spells, dances, often by masked people, prayers with sacrifices, amulets, soul hunt in trance, change of names, magic transfer of disease to animals or plants, the use of fetishes and medicine bundles. Mutilation, painting, and tattooing are used as magic therapeutics or prophylaxis.

Urine and saliva as medicaments are undoubtedly of magic origin. While primitive drugs in general are specific for one disease, these two are clearly panaceas, i.e., drugs that cure all diseases. The dream of a panacea fills human thought from its beginnings to the Enlightenment. Urine is a panacea from Herodot to Lemery, spittle from the Bible to Brera.

In order to reach a real understanding of primitive therapeutics, it is necessary to transgress the description of their naturalistic as well as supernaturalistic methods. The real difference between these therapeutics and ours is not a matter of effectiveness. The latter was, till a hundred years ago, probably not very different in both medicines. One should never have illusions about the effectiveness of primitive as well as of other historical therapeutics. The real difference is based on the fact that primitives use the same naturalistic elements, which we still use, merely as parts of a magico-religious system oriented toward the supernatural in cause and effect. This system does not use our categories and does not differentiate, for example, between therapeutics and diagnosis or prognosis. The divinatory diagnosis is at the same time treatment. Primitive therapeutics is essentially a more or less grandiose magico-religious show in which mechanistic elements are integrated. In this show, sucking as a means of eliminating the supernatural principle of disease very often plays a central role. In this system profane and magico-religious methods are indissolubly linked. It is a system based not primarily on experience, not to mention experiment, but on holy traditions or religious intuition. This system is very conservative. A relatively rapid and strong effect is aimed at. As this treatment is mostly directed against one particular disease-producing demon, it is in a way "specific."

A healing ceremony with the North American Navajo Indians proceeds as follows: the medicine man (called singer by them) comes on the eve of the treatment to the house of the sick and speaks some prayers. The next morning the hut is cleaned, a new fire lighted and a so-called bull roarer, a sacred rattle, activated. All participants —patient, relatives, and medicine man—wash and take an emetic. With eagle feathers the singer symbolically brushes the evil away from the patient. All jump over the fire, all sweat. Each step of this ceremony is accompanied by holy songs and prayers. Then the hut is fumigated, and there is singing again. This continues for four days, and ritual baths, sacrifices, and sand painting appear as elements in the course of the treatment.

The magic nature of many of these methods has often been overlooked because they are effective, and we identify erroneously the scientifically naturalistic with the effective. The magic nature of certain drugs is furthermore overlooked because they are used quite rationally with us. Yet it is possible to find out rather rapidly the actual meaning of a therapeutic procedure if, for example, it is only effective if it is paid for. This is an old magic point of view which is defended today only by some psychotherapeutic sects. We might mention here that even primitive therapeutics is sometimes very costly.

It is equally not customary among us to assume that the effect of a drug is the same whether it is taken by the patient himself or the medicine man or a relative. From the point of view of the primitive it is irrelevant whether the drug is effective in our sense or not. In both cases for him the magic strength of the drug, its symbolic value, is decisive. It is typical for the peculiarities of primitive therapeutics that in collecting and preparing drugs certain ceremonies are prescribed. Drugs are either inherited or bought or dreamed or sometimes discovered. A great many primitive drugs have been taken over by white men. Drugs whose effect is interpreted by the ancient hot and cold dichotomy have probably been taken over by primitives from the whites.

Where really lie the origins of drugs, especially of the effective ones? Unfortunately we can only formulate hypotheses on this problem. The assumption of an original empiricism which later was submerged by magic, i.e., the assumption that some people tried all existing herbs in all diseases, is not very convincing, even if one assumes that only herbs with a special taste were taken into consideration. This theory is probably the consequence of the old illusion that each effective action is founded on or has been founded by rational thought and therefore is effective. Another hypothesis is that the first drugs were found by instinct, a somewhat vague notion that does not lead us very far.

It is most likely that many therapeutic actions never become conscious but remain on the level of the habitual. Certainly the one or the other thing is also learned from experience. But if theories do exist, it seems that the earliest theories were of a magic nature. These magic theories have led to an inflation of the pharmacopoeia with many ineffective substances. Empirical things have been added too. The victory of the rational has come relatively late. Thereafter the magic drugs have been rationalized somehow.

A specific kind of "treatment" is the killing of the sick which is observed in some primitive tribes. So far no connection between this cruel custom and other technological or ideological elements of the respective culture has been found. It cannot be overlooked that the mass killing of sick people was practiced even in civilized Europe only thirty years ago. Frequently primitives refuse to treat the incurable, a point of view that even in our medicine was not regarded as unethical up to the eighteenth century and can be found in all medicines whether Greek, Hindu, or Chinese.

Suicide of the incurable is not rare either. Certain forms of primitive therapeutics impress us rather as a conscious or unconscious punishment of the sick than as treatment. This impression returns over and over again in the course of history.

One peculiarity of primitive therapeutics is a kind of specialization, which is not based on a plentitude of knowledge, like our specialization, but on a lack of knowledge. One medicine man always knows only a few ceremonies, and the methods connected with them, which are directed against a specific disease or disease demon and which are inherited. The buying of such secret knowledge is so expensive that it is realized only rarely.

Having discussed some basic traits of primitive therapeutics, we will take up several details. The pharmacopoeia of primitives is in general surprisingly large. It is true, a very sizable percentage are ineffective. Not rarely, primitive pharmacopoeias contain the so-called Dreckapotheke, i.e., excrements of men and animals. Primitives know, on the other hand, numerous curative plants which are either collected or even planted and among which some, on account of their effectiveness, are used even today. I mention here only strychnine, picrotoxin, aconite, physostigmine, strophanthin, which originate from so-called savages. The same holds for quinine, emetine, cocaine, and lobelia. Tobacco, too, was originally a drug. Digitalis and ergot derive from the primitive layers of our own culture. Only twenty years ago a drug gained from the primitive herb rauwolfia opened a whole new field in pharmacotherapy, the psychopharmaceuticals. Till recently primitive drugs like eucalyptus, podophylline, sarsaparilla, acacia, copaiba, guaiac, perubalm and tolubalm, and a large number of primitive emetics, diuretics, purgatives, expectorants, anthelmintics, narcotics, abortives, and supposedly anticonceptual drugs were used.

The use of animal parts was not limited to excrements, but also fat (e.g., of the tiger), organs (like the liver), bones (in China sold under the name of dragon bones, actually fossil bones), the so-called bezoar, parts of toads, human blood, human flesh, and human spittle (in Europe used till the nineteenth century!) play a not inconsiderable role. Minerals were used less by the primitives. Yet we encounter the use of sulfur, copper, silicates, sodium chlorate, soda, and saltpeter. In general the effect was not attributed to an impersonal natural quality of the drug but to a magic principle in the drug or in the prescribing medicine man.

The number of drugs known in one particular tribe varies very much. In general it would be from about 100 to 200 medicaments, but in some tribes many more, in others many less are known. The magic element, i.e., the magic spell, can be so overwhelming in the curative ritual that no drugs at all are used. There can also be a natural lack of drugs. The absence of drugs is reported from Melanesia and the Arctics, also from the North American Mojave and Hawasupai, the South American Yagua, the Indian Toda, and the African Dama. The Maori of New Zealand are supposed to have learned the use of drugs only from the white invaders.

Clysters are extremely popular, especially in Africa and South America. They are used with the same enthusiasm as in our own seventeenth century. The keeping of a special diet is not rare. In the Hippocratic book on old medicine, diet is spoken of as something very old, the source of medicine, derived from experience. Observations of primitives rather indicate that diet is not always of rational origin, but was magic, to be rationalized only later. A diet can very easily be generated by fasting for visionary dreams. It is significant that there is a diet among the Cherokee Indians of North America that is kept only during daytime, because there are taboos that are obeyed only during daytime. During the night the patient does not keep the diet.

Sweat baths are very widely known and occur with or without supernatural representations. Massage is also popular, especially in Melanesia; there is no doubt that massage here was developed to drive out the disease demon. Therefore a massage movement is centrifugal and not, as with us, centripetal. The very frequently used cupping could be derived from the sucking out of a magic foreign body, the classic rite of primitive medicine. Certain techniques of bloodletting, like the use of miniature bows and arrows, point toward magic origins. Even vaccinations, like that against snakebite, probably have supernaturalistic foundations. Otherwise it would not be understandable why, for example, in Liberia the tourniquet is replaced by a white line.

Surgery is developed only weakly. It consists primarily in wound treatment, in which the magic spells play a great role. The same holds for the treatment of fractures. Incisions are rare. Amputations are extremely rare and reported only from East Africa and Polynesia. But some primitives practice such heroic operations as caesarean section or trepanation. Only magic origins could explain the contradiction between the existence of such very complicated surgical manipulations and the total absence of such practices in other tribes.

Even in the framework of the magic there is local and general treatment. As primitives are not acquainted with our body-soul dualism, specific mental disease or specific psychotherapy is rarely assumed.

We have already mentioned the strictly magic techniques like spells, trance, transference, amulets, change of name. The medicine man, a master of the supernatural, has at his disposal certain paraphernalia like rattles, drums, containers of magic substances. In general, he inherits his office from his father or uncle. Often unusual experiences like visions, podalic birth, being struck by lightning, or surviving a deadly disease destined him to become a medicine man.

As possession by a demon is one of the main causes of disease with primitives, healing ceremonies are very often exorcisms. With the Ga of the African west coast exorcism takes, according to Margaret J. Field, the following course:

"The patient sits naked on a special stool in the bush and holds on his head a vessel full of medicinal leaves and water. Two medicine men with six apprentices drum and sing monotonous invitations to the ghost, to leave the patient. The patient moves unsteadily. He appears more and more intoxicated (i.e., he is afterward amnestic). Eventually the ghost leaves him, the patient runs crying into the bush and, after a purification ceremony, is sent home."

From our point of view the basic element in primitive therapeutics is, in spite of drugs and physiotherapy, psychotherapeutic procedures. Eugene Bleuler said in his *Autistic Thought* rightly: "Primitive medicine is, in spite of the tangible nature of the used magic substances, psychological; it could only be effective by way of suggestion, and the whole procedure of how the one conquers the other, is only a play of two psyches." Besides suggestion, the ritual of confessing plays a very important role in primitive therapy. Both psychological forces are used today consciously or unconsciously very frequently in our medicine.

It is difficult to evaluate the actual value of primitive therapeutics. Two things are certain: Primitives are not easily inclined to give up their traditions. Many Western observers have judged the results of primitive therapeutics rather favorably, and it is quite possible that this view was justifiable before the appearance of infectious disease in these isolated groups.

In primitive societies therapeutics is practiced not only by single laymen or professional medicine men or medicine women, but frequently in medicine societies (e.g., with the North American Zuni or Ojibwa). And even if there is no official society, almost always a number of relatives or neighbors gather around the medicine man and his patient and participate in the curative procedure. Parallels with modern group therapy are obvious.

The physician of today differs from the medicine man insofar as he tries (with the exception of a small minority which despises science) to think and to act scientifically. The attitude of the patient is very different. Even in the most civilized countries, many look at physicians as "magicians." This tendency is reinforced by the idle talk of "miracle drugs" or "second reality." Elements of primitive medicine thus survive in different areas of medicine, not just in the area of effective vegetable drugs.

II

Egyptian Therapeutics

THE MEDICINE of early man and the primitives is followed by a medicine of the early civilizations which is called "archaic medicine." Technological, ideological, and sociological changes led from nomadic tribes to empires based on agriculture, from the nonliterate prehistoric tribes to people having books. Therewith history starts, and in medicine subjective and objective changes are clearly visible. We know of such archaic medicine in Egypt, Mesopotamia, India, China, Persia, Israel, Phoenicia, Crete, with the old Etruscans, Mexicans, Peruvians, and elsewhere. In the framework of this book we have to limit ourselves to a description of the therapeutics in Egyptian archaic medicine as a model of all others. These therapeutics are, of course, objectively symptomatic.

The Egyptian medical papyri which were written mostly in the second millennium B.C. are, together with Mesopotamian clay tablets, the oldest medical documents we know. They probably often reflect medical ideas and experiences that are much older, i.e., go back to the beginning of the fourth millennium B.C.

Egyptian medicine is, like all areas of life in Egypt, dominated by the supernatural. This is obvious when priests or magicians treat sick people. But even so-called doctors have been either priests or very close to the priestly caste, very similar in this respect to medieval physicians. Consequently, in every kind of treatment prayer, spell, or conjuration plays an important role. Not accidentally the *Papyrus Ebers,* probably the richest medical document from Egypt at our disposal, begins with three such formulas, and several prescriptions in the same papyrus contain other conjurations of supernatural forces.

Yet the important element in Egyptian medicine is not the supernaturalistic, well known from primitive medicine, but the naturalistic empirical element, which is much stronger here than in primitive medicine, where subjectively supernaturalistic ideas, objectively psychotherapeutics, prevail. There are medical papyri which contain almost no spells. Aside from supernaturalistic ideas the medical papyri are based on naturalistic theories, naturalistic descriptions of disease, and naturalistic methods of treatment. Only the latter will be dealt with here in detail.

To illustrate Egyptian therapeutics we give here a typical passage from the *Papyrus Ebers:*

"a) If you examine a man with an obstruction of his stomach and if he vomits with pain, he suffers like a sh.t.

"Then you should say: this is a collection of excrement which has not yet solidified.

"b) Then you should give him a potion: figs ⅛; milk ¹⁄₁₆; fruits of the sycamores ⅛. Let this mixture stand during the night in sweet beer 10 ro, filter it and let it be drunk very, very often so that he gets again healthy immediately."

Drug therapeutics seems to have been in the center of Egyptian medicine. Some Egyptian medical books (papyri) consist almost exclusively of prescriptions. The *Papyrus Ebers,* for example, contains 800. For the Egyptians these prescriptions were partly not human inventions, but the inventions of gods. It is remarkable that the form of the Egyptian prescription is the same that we still use (in case we do write prescriptions, which has become rather rare). The old Egyptian prescription also consists of three parts: (1) enumeration of the drugs, (2) instructions for the apothecary (or, as there were no apothecaries in Egypt, the doctor) on how to prepare the remedy, (3) instructions for the patient on how to take the remedy. First, just as in our own prescriptions, are enumerated the effective substances, the so-called basis, then the constituent, i.e., the medium for the effective substances (in general, oil, water, grease, or beer). It is notable that, in the prescriptions, exact measures are given. Unfortunately the Egyptologists have not yet agreed in their translation.

In general the difficulties for the translator of this dead language are great. Numerous drugs mentioned in the prescriptions either have not been identified up to this day, or are interpreted differently by different translators. External as well as internal remedies are prescribed. Polypharmacy, i.e., the prescription of numerous substances in one single formula, is one of the most striking and one of the least attractive characteristics of Egyptian therapeutics.

Among the drugs, substances of plant origin prevail. Among these above all are cathartics like ricinus, coloquint, senna. Ricinus was also used, as today, as a cosmetic; like garlic, it is one of those great panaceas that always return: in Dioskorides, in the Middle Ages, today. Emphasis on cathartics is understandable in a medicine in which theoretically the gastrointestinal tract, especially the anus, is the main seat of disease. Effective vermifuges, like pomegranate, were known. Vermifuges were for thousands of years to come of great practical importance. Other plants used by Egyptians are hyoscyamus, vermouth, juniper, mustard, turpentine, scilla, as a cough medicine and emetic. In addition many worthless substances, like sawdust, were used. A great many things prescribed would be regarded today as pure kitchen products, such as oil, beans, onions, honey, figs, barley, wheat, celery, and pistachio. It is not entirely certain but very likely that opium preparations were prescribed.

Drugs from the animal kingdom were extremely numerous too. Everything the ox can deliver was used as a medicament: his meat, his gall, etc. Also the gall of the turtle or the organs of other animals, like the uterus of cats, were frequently employed. Very popular was fat of the hippopotamus, of the antelope, of the ass, the crocodile, or the goose. Eggs of ravens or geese were medicaments as well as bones or horns of gazelles. Woman's milk played the therapeutic role it continued to play up to the eighteenth century. The so-called Dreckapotheke, such as excrements of birds, of children, is of course not lacking. That liver is prescribed for night blindness is perhaps an accident, perhaps more. Names in prescriptions, like "ass' head," "mouse tail," have to be handled with caution. Apparently it is not the real thing, but a comparative name for plants, as our own "snapdragon."

Eventually minerals were used, like copper, iron oxide, sodium carbonate, sulfur, antimony, zinc oxide, especially in ointments. Salves were used not only in skin diseases but also in eye diseases, which apparently even then were very frequent in Egypt. Medicaments were given in the form of decoctions, pills, powders, clysters, anal suppositories. The same drugs are prescribed over and over again for very different diseases. The bad panacea habit seems already in existence. Many medicaments are, as mentioned, not identified even today. The prevalence of cathartics and clysters (the *Papyrus Ebers* starts with no less than forty cathartic prescriptions) would be even easier to understand if the old Egyptians had had a humoral pathology like the Greeks. But we lack evidence for this. The interpretation of an inflammation of the eyes as a sign of putrefying phlegm in the abdomen points perhaps in this direction. There is no doubt that the Greeks took over many Egyptian drugs and probably also some

Egyptian theories. It is, on the other hand, surprising that in the Egyptian therapeutic literature, at least as far as we know it, diet in the Greek sense (which was the central element in Greek medicine) plays no role—if we do not want to regard the use of kitchen vegetables like beans, onions, and figs, as medicaments, as a form of diet. This interpretation would seem to be a little overdrawn.

Very remarkable is that, in the Egyptian therapeutic literature, the otherwise universally popular bloodletting is not mentioned. This is all the more surprising as the Egyptian physiology and pathology of the human body, which mirrors the canal system of the country, would have been ideal for rationalizing such a practice. Passing mention might be made of the fact that some papyri, particularly the *Papyrus Ebers,* also contain products against insect plagues or mice or other parasites.

Respect for Egyptian surgery has greatly increased since the *Papyrus Smith* has been found. A typical surgical case from the *Papyrus Smith* is the following: "Information on a wound at the top of a brow.

"If you examine a man with a wound on the top of his brow, which goes to the bone, then you should palpate the wound and tie it together with a thread.

"Then you should say: 'One with a wound on the top of his brow. A disease which I will treat.'

"After having sewed the wound, you should put on the wound raw flesh on the first day. If you find that the suture has changed place, then you should put on two bandages. Treat him with oil and honey every day till he is better.

"What concerns the two bandages from cloth.

"They are two strips of cloth which one puts at the lips of a gaping wound in order to put one margin of the wound to the other."

Of course this surgery, though utilizing the hot iron and the knife, is, like all surgery up to the nineteenth century, above all wound surgery. The *Papyrus Smith* discusses exclusively the treatment of wounds and fractures with salves, plasters, and splints. The surgical chapters of the *Papyrus Ebers* indicate a more active attitude in the case of swollen lymph nodes, hernia, atheromas, abscesses, and aneurysms. Nevertheless it seems legitimate to characterize Egyptian surgery and Egyptian medicine as a surgery and medicine that were relatively nonaggressive and relied to a large extent on the natural healing process, whether this notion was already theoretically developed or not.

Egyptian papyri, especially the *Papyrus Smith,* contain not rarely the refusal of treatment of incurables, mentioned in the chapter on primitive medicine. On the other hand, in other places, e.g., in the *Papyrus Ebers,* there is a direct order not to abandon the sick. This produces the impression, which is confirmed by later materials, that the rule not to treat the incurable was ethically absolutely legitimate up to the eighteenth century but was not generally applied.

III

Hippocratic Therapeutics

THE OLDEST known extensive documents concerning Greek medicine are the so-called Hippocratic writings from the fifth and fourth centuries B.C.* This body of literature is a tremendous turning point in the history of medicine in general and in the history of therapeutics in particular. The secularization which in archaic medicine, like the Egyptian, only begins is here completely adopted, whether the writings are influenced by the school of Cos or by the school of Cnidos. This is very clearly illustrated by the change in meaning of the word "pharmakon." In Homer, pharmakon still is a magic substance (in the sense of remedy as well as of poison); in Hesiod, in the eighth century B.C., it is already a natural substance. In the Hippocratic writings it is either a remedy (possibly the element of a diet) or a drug or a cathartic. The fact that the notion of cathartic is so pervasive points toward magic origins which are now rationalized by humoral pathology † and humoral therapeutics. The same drugs now no longer drive out evil spirits from vessels or intestines or lungs or the bladder or nose, but produce a "derivation" or "revulsion" of bad humors. The practitioners are no longer magicians or priests, but craftsmen.

Hippocratic therapeutics are based on an entirely new concept of disease. Disease is no longer an individual, is not regarded ontologically, is not a secularized demon. Disease is now a changed state of the body. Therefore, one does not treat "the disease" but the state of the sick patient. This presupposes individualization of the methods. The Hippocratic method of treating the patient and not the disease is at the same time wisdom and the consequence of medical ignorance. Since the Greeks medicine has oscillated between this Hippocratic and the so-called ontological method of treating disease. Even if the Hippocratic physicians would have tried to treat "the disease," as we do today in certain cases to a certain extent, they

---

* We speak here of "Hippocratic writings" and not of the writings of Hippocrates, because it seems useless to participate in the now two-millennia-old discussion of whether the writings that have been handed down under the name of Hippocrates are authentic or not.

† Humoral pathology explains diseases as the disturbance of the balance and the composition of the four humors: blood, yellow bile, black bile, and phlegm, of which supposedly the body is composed. Humoral therapy consists of measures destined to reestablish the equilibrium of the four humors.

could not have been successful in view of their ignorance of diseases. They knew only symptoms. To treat the sick patient was possible to them. This largely symptomatic treatment of the patient is based on the assumption of the healing power of nature, which works in the patient and tends toward a reestablishment of his health. This power can be observed, e.g., in wound healing or fracture healing. These tendencies of nature are mostly interpreted in the sense of humoral pathology, i.e., as a so-called coction. Self-healing is usually brought about by a crisis. These ideas are, of course, vitalistic. The physician is no longer the primitive magician, but plays the more modest but more useful role of a servant ("minister," in Latin) of nature.

Out of this spirit grows the often repeated and often not sufficiently respected Hippocratic slogan that the physician is supposed to be useful or at least not to do harm, a slogan equally great as a technical rule and as the expression of rational ethics. This is certainly one of the most important elements of Hippocratic medicine.

The so-called healing power of nature has, in the later course of history, played an official role from Sydenham through Stahl to Virchow. Today it has become almost exclusively a slogan of the so-called nature healers, i.e., insufficiently trained healing practitioners who can be subjectively honest or dishonest. These people have also preserved the theories of the cleaning of humors, i.e., the fossils of ancient official medicine. We too assume a kind of healing power of nature, but no longer in the primitive animistic sense, but in a scientific sense of curative, more precisely defined and measurable reactions and regulations of the body such as the formation of immunity and mobilization of hormones.

In the disease theories of the ancients, especially those following the school of Cos, disease is located in the whole body. The Cnidian school was apparently more localistic. The assumption of the generalized nature of disease makes the treatment of the whole body necessary. Therefore the popularity of cathartics. It is noticeable that even with those physicians of Greco-Roman civilization who did not follow humoral pathology but some kind of a pathology of solids, treatment was general, not localistic. If one subscribes to the theory of the healing power of nature, it is logical to regard fever as a therapeutic. The Greek physician Rufos even asked for artificial fever. Also regarded as therapeutics are bleeding hemorrhoids and menstruation. Based, too, on this theory is the creation of blisters or artificial ulcers ("fontanelles") to derive, or draw out, the bad humors. This is thought to complete the usual methods of derivation (clysters, bleeding, vomiting, sweating, burning, etc.) and was unfortunately practiced up into the nineteenth century. The seton is in antiquity known only to veterinary medicine, where we call it rowel. In human medicine it appears only in Salerno.

In order to gain a concrete picture of Hippocratic therapeutics, it is probably best to study briefly the famous Hippocratic treatise on diet in acute diseases. The acute diseases—i.e., pleurisy, pneumonia, brain inflammation, burning fever—were those with which the ancient physicians had to deal primarily. The author of the treatise belongs without doubt to the school of Cos, from which the historical Hippocrates originated. He turns, in the beginning, against the competing school of Cnidos, which, in the case of acute diseases, only evacuates and gives some milk diet, but not enough diet in the sense of a general arrangement of daily life. His own practice is based above all on barley gruel (ptisane). Two thirds of the book deal with this, so that one could almost call it a book on barley gruel. In addition, the author gives lots of fluids, above all honey water (hydromel) or honey water with vinegar (oxymel), more rarely wine and almost never water. After the crisis, which supposedly occurs on the seventh day, he gives solid food. If barley gruel "gets stuck," e.g., if the sputum does not soften in pneumonia, he gives a clyster or bleeds; otherwise there is danger of worsening of the condition. In pain in the chest he recommends hot water bottles, hot sponges, hot bags and, if no improvement occurs, bloodletting. In pain in the lower abdomen he prescribes the drastic helleborus or euphorbia.

The author is not in favor of fasting at the beginning of the disease, even less so of cutting liquids. In general one should keep the usual rhythm of meals (such who eat once a day should continue eating once a day; such who eat twice a day should eat twice a day). Each change of rhythm is dangerous even in the healthy. This importance of habit is also emphasized later on by Erasistratus and Galen. The same opinion is uttered in the Hippocratic treatise on ancient medicine. One should let the patients sleep (there were ancient schools which disturbed sleep), and if they cannot sleep, one should let them walk a little.

After a few days one could start fasting; but after fasting one should be very cautious before returning to normal food. All change is dangerous, such as from flat cakes to bread, from wine to water. The author discusses the advantage of different beverages (wine, hydromel, oxymel) and baths, where one should individualize.

The second part of the treatise was regarded in ancient times already as nonauthentic. It does not contain anything basically new. It recommends again diet, bloodletting, cathartics and emetics, expectorants, and ass' milk. It discusses the poor digestibility of certain foods like garlic, cheese, leguminous plants, and certain meats. It recommends cantharides in dropsy and copper in eye diseases.

This book belongs to those Hippocratic writings that are based exclusively on humoral pathology, i.e., above all on the pathology of gall (bile) and phlegm. This is the reason why evacuation and cathartics are so important to the author. If we look at the many minutiae of his dietary arrangements, we cannot say that they were necessary, but it is quite possible that they had a psychotherapeutic value and made unnecessary the giving of drugs which is obligatory with us. Altogether a patient was probably not in bad hands with a Hippocratic therapist of this kind.

Not only in the above-analyzed treatise of the Corpus Hippocraticum on acute diseases is diet in the center of therapeutics. This holds true for the majority of Hippocratic writings. One of them, that on ancient medicine, derives the whole medical art directly from diet. Barbarians supposedly had no diet! Dietary prescriptions are not limited to extensive catalogues of food, but include the prescription of several kinds of bodily exercise, walking, etc. Only later (with Aretaios) does climate become an element of these dietetic prescriptions.

Besides diet and physiotherapeutics the Hippocratic physician used about 250 medicinal plants. Only few remedies came from the animal kingdom. These drugs are above all cathartics, the most powerful of which is helleborus, also effective in insanity; in addition are emetics, diuretics, warming remedies. Some Hippocratic writings are more inclined to prescribe drugs than others, e.g., *De affectionibus*. This book refers frequently to a lost book of the Hippocratic collection on drugs. The book *De morbis* recommends in pneumonia expectorants like sage, in fevers cooling remedies, in night blindness liver. In hysteria bad-smelling remedies are supposed to drive the migrating uterus back in its place or good smells from below are supposed to entice it to return. In prolapse of the uterus the opposite procedure is recommended. Baths are therapeutically very important. The Hippocratic writings do not very often recommend the use of bloodletting.

The Hippocratic writings contain several excellent books on surgery, a surgery that is, of course, like all surgery till 150 year ago, far more conservative than ours. These writings deal with the reposition of luxated articulations and the treatment of fractures and wounds. For the treatment of wounds several bandages are described. Here we find the greatest number of prescriptions in the Hippocratic corpus. Celsus and medieval treatises show the same abundance of prescriptions in the surgical chapters. The prescriptions are ointments for wounds or for cleaning the uterus. The surgical writings of the Corpus Hippocraticum discuss also trepanation in skull trauma and treatment of hemorrhoids with the hot iron, by cutting or caustic salves. A speculum for the anus is known. Anal fistula is treated with the thread method. In difficult obstetric cases embryotomy is recommended. Contraceptives are also known.

Besides a craftsman-scientific medicine the Greeks also had religious medicine in the temples of the god Asklepios, which were erected simultaneously with the writing of the Hippocratic treatises. Here, as before in the temples of Imhotep in Egypt or later in Christian temples, curative sleep was practiced. The patient slept in the temple and was cured during his sleep by the god. It is probably symbolic for the predilection of the Greeks for hygiene and panaceas that among the seven mythical children of Asklepios and his wife, Epione, we find a goddess Hygeia as well as a goddess Panakeia. While the physician-craftsmen primarily served a thin upper class, religious medicine took care of much larger segments of the population.

IV

From the Alexandrians to Dioskorides

AMONG THE successors of Hippocrates, the so-called dogmatists (they follow the dogma of the master), an activation of therapeutics is quite visible. The most famous of them, Diokles of Karystos (about 360 B.C.), continues the dietary prescriptions of the teacher, but simultaneously he writes the first Greek herbal and a number of other treatises on pharmaca and poisons.

After the beginning of the third pre-Christian century the center of Greek medicine is located for several centuries in Alexandria, the North African foundation of Alexander the Great. Famous and anatomically competent Alexandrian physicians like Herophilos and Erasistratus differ in many respects from Hippocrates, among other things through an activation of therapeutics. Herophilos, who is still a humoral pathologist, is a great friend of medicaments. He calls drugs "the hands of the gods" and is, as far as bloodletting is concerned, far more active than the Hippocratists. His younger contemporary, Erasistratus (about 310–250 B.C.), who subscribes to a pathology of the solids, opposes too much bleeding and insists on the value of diet. He is nevertheless a rather aggressive therapist.

An anecdote concerning Erasistratus shows how familiar Greek clinicians were with psychosomatic situations. King Seleukos called Erasistratus because his son from a first marriage, Antiochus, was pining away for unknown reasons. Erasistratus diagnosed suffering from unfulfilled love. He found as the cause the stepmother of Antiochus, Stratonike, as she was the only woman who produced in Antiochus by her presence a quickened pulse, change of complexion, and sweating.

The so-called sect of empiricists played a great role in Alexandrian medicine. Their attitude toward bloodletting was less positive than that of Herophilos and his disciples. But they pleaded for giving drugs. The use of opium was propagated above all by the empiricist Herakleides. Characteristic for the addiction to drugs in Alexandria is that theriac, a panacea used up to the nineteenth century, which always was composed of dozens of substances, is probably an Alexandrian invention. The pharmacopoeia of the Alexandrians was much larger than the Hippocratic one, as Alexander and his men brought back a great number of drugs from the Orient. Very important is also the great progress in surgery achieved in Alexandria.

Occasionally the Hippocratic books mention experience in a laudatory way, but the first aphorism calls it fallacious. The Hippocratic books contain quite a few empirical facts. But it is only in the third century that in Alexandria, in connection with skeptic philosophy, a school of men arise who, disgusted with dogmatism and rationalism, call themselves empiricists and claim to base their medicine exclusively on experience and really are the first to analyze the problem. But what really is "therapeutic experience"?

In the course of history probably most physicians have claimed that experience is at least partially the basis of their therapeutics. This sounds very simple and convincing. In reality therapeutic experience is something far more complicated and problematic. Jaccoud said rightly, "Let's not forget, seeing is not observing." Actually the therapeutics of most physicians are dependent on traditions and authority, and rarely is therapeutic faith changed by actual experience. Lasagna has shown that physicians believe more in the textbook than in their own experience! Besides prejudice, a great number of other factors can falsify actual experience. The best known experiential error is the "post hoc, propter hoc" fallacy which in therapeutics has played a devastating role. There are, of course, a number of valuable drugs and measures that have grown out of experience, but most things that have been presented in the course of the millennia as experience were pseudoexperience, or "false experience" as Johann Georg Zimmermann in his book about experience in medicine called it. Most of the so-called empiricists were pseudo-empiricists. Petersen speaks of "superficial and sanguine application of the law of casuality, little respect for exact conclusions, firm belief in unproven presuppositions and lack in method and skepsis" in many empirical therapists. Martini calls this "naïve experience" which is poorly controlled and generalizes single events.

If most of older experience were not pseudoexperience, the whole horrifying history of therapeutics, its bloodletting vampirism, its polypharmacy, its highly toxic drugs, its panaceas, its sudden changes from one method to the opposite, its claim of experience as the basis for two opposite methods, etc., etc.—this all would be unthinkable. In view of this situation it is not a very good idea to present the history of therapeutics simply as a history of "empiricism versus rationalism," as Petersen did.

In order to collect real experience in therapeutics, a certain number of methods of objectivation are necessary which complete or replace the all too subjective, forgetful or autistic judgment of the observer. Such methods have developed only very slowly.

The fate of the empiricists, who ended soon in a dead end and were forgotten, shows that valuable theories concerning experience are not equivalent to the actual acquisition of valid experiences. The empiricists opposed the dogmatists, who based their therapeutics primarily on theories and intended to build upon their own experience, to use inherited experience and analogy-conclusions. With this so-called tripos they did not go very far. And their most valuable cognizances—i.e., that experiences, in order to be valid, have to be repeated frequently and that also negative results have to be reported—were completely forgotten shortly after their appearance.

During the time of Hippocrates physicians collected their drugs themselves and also prepared them. At the time of the botanist Theophrastus (he died in 287 B.C.), a special profession of drug collectors (rhizotomoi) developed. Later there existed also large (emporoi) and small (kapeloi) drug dealers. The latter were not esteemed very highly, nor were a sort of quacks who were very much occupied with drugs, the pharmakopoloi. Among the physicians of Alexandria some seem to have specialized in the knowledge and preparation of drugs, i.e., their activity was very similar to that of our apothecaries of the past. The expression "Apotheke" was used in classic antiquity, but originally in the meaning of the storeroom for drugs, which every physician had in his office. Those processing drugs, physicians and nonphysicians, used, of course, a number of instruments like hand mills, mortars, sieves, balances, which have been found in excavations.

In the work of Asklepiades (who lived around 100–50 B.C.) we find a reaction against therapeutic overactivity. He was the first successful Greek physician in Rome. He influenced strongly the so-called methodists. Asklepiades was an anti-Hippocratist and a mechanist. He opposed the theory of the healing force of nature and of crises. He characterized Hippocratic medicine as a long wait for death and rejected humoral pathology. Medicine, he said in a rather quackish way, should act "fast, with certainty and agreeably" (*cito, tuto, iucunde*). Yet actually his practice was very sensible. He condemned the overuse of drugs (emetics, cathartics, specifics). He felt that too many drugs will exert harmful stimuli on the body. In this respect the methodists followed him. He rarely used bloodletting and clysters. On this point the methodists did not follow him insofar as in their so-called status strictus they recommended bleeding on the opposite side. The therapeutics of Asklepiades consisted primarily in prevention, or diet with a lot of fasting, baths, wine, and music. He was such a great friend of baths that his contemporaries called him the "water doctor," and he appears to us as one of the fathers of physical therapy. He also recommended movement, not only in the healthy, but as an excellent remedy. Suggestions of motion therapy are found in Hippocrates. Asklepiades felt that traveling was very good for soul and body. He knew tracheotomy. His recommendation to let the patient stay awake and thirst in fever is less meritorious. Opinions on the value of bed rest have changed continuously in the history of therapeutics. Asklepiades also very much favored massage, particularly the rubbing of the vertebral column, so that he could also be regarded as the precursor of certain modern physiotherapeutic sects. Asklepiades was, in summary, through his expectative practice, which does not correspond to his grandiloquent activistic theory, without any doubt a very important reformer of ancient therapeutics.

The methodists, theoretically rather dull with their "status strictus" and "status laxus" as the only two disease causes, continued in general the work of Asklepiades. They too did not think very highly of vomiting and evacuation. They emphasized particularly the so-called metasyncritic treatment, i.e., a treatment that changes the reaction of the total body. The frequent use of leeches originated supposedly with the methodist Themison. We will later give a concrete example of methodist therapy, when discussing a chapter from Soranos. Many methodists were not able to defend the reforms of Asklepiades.

After Asklepiades, Greek medicine entered more and more in Rome. The Romans themselves were not creative in the field of medicine, although their baths, their water supplies, and their sewerages were outstanding. Aulus Cornelius Celsus (born about 35 B.C., died about A.D. 50) wrote a large encyclopedia, but only the medical part *De medicina libri octo* has survived. The medical contemporaries of Celsus, who probably was no physician but a layman, apparently took no notice of him. Celsus became really famous in medicine

only during the Renaissance, when his *De medicina libri octo* formed
an excellent compendium of old medicine, written in very pure
and clear Latin. As a compendium Celsus remains interesting for
the historian. A comparison of the therapeutic methods described
by him with those we have found in the Hippocratic writings shows
us the evolution of Greek medicine from 400 to 1 B.C., an evolution
about which otherwise we know very little.

Celsus subdivides medicine into three great divisions: diet (in the
largest sense of the word, including physiotherapy), pharmacy, and
surgery. It is typical that he begins his book with rules for the
healthy. Then he reviews the different curative methods: bleeding,
cupping, evacuation, vomiting, rubbing, passive movement, fasting, sweating, and diet (in the sense of regulation of food intake).
The influences of the Hippocratic writings and of Asklepiades are
very obvious. Many dangerous diseases are, according to Celsus, cured
simply by a rest and fasting.

Celsus deals extensively with the treatment of general diseases. He
begins with the treatment of fever. Here he recommends evacuation,
bleeding, and fasting. It is interesting that he insists that the sick
should be kept free from worries. In treating exhaustion he mentions
nourishing clysters. In dropsy he prescribes strict abstention from
liquid, diuretics, and puncture of the abdomen. Against phthisis he
recommends change of climate, sleeping, milk, and artificial ulcers,
which are also suggested in the Hippocratic writings. He treats epilepsy
with diet, bleeding, and cathartics; he opposes the habit of letting
the patient drink, in this disease, the blood of gladiators, but is in
favor of burning the occiput. Jaundice, leprosy, and apoplexy, which
are rather different, are nevertheless all treated with diet, bleeding,
and cathartics.

In the next part of the book, where Celsus discusses the treatment of local diseases, he enumerates them in the classic sequence
"a capite ad calcem" (from head to foot). Again we encounter the
old triad: diet, bleeding, and cathartics, whether he deals with a
headache or pneumonia. In so-called lientery he recommends iron
waters and diuretics, in kidney disease a salt-free diet. In diseases of
the hip joint he prescribes derivative ulcers, which he favors in general. The catalogue of drugs and prescriptions in the book of Celsus
shows the same tendency as the Hippocratic writings, i.e., to use

such substances especially in surgery. It is interesting that he recommends arsenical salves for cauterizing cancer. Mithridaticum, the older brother of theriac, contains with him thirty-six substances. He knows a soporific medicine composed of opium and mandragora.

In the field of wound treatment Celsus is, as in all surgery, strongly influenced by Alexandrian examples. He recommends the suturing of fresh wounds and ligature against bleeding. He prescribes milk against poison. Treating so-called ulcers, he makes a statement that cancer gets worse through burning and cutting; nevertheless he later describes an operation for carcinoma of the penis. In scabies he uses a sulfur ointment. In ophthalmology he knows the operation of cataract with the needle, and also the use of the blood of swallows in eye diseases and of liver in hemeralopy. He describes plastic operations of the ears and the prepuce. To remove hemorrhoids, which are regarded by humoral pathologists as very useful, he deems a dangerous enterprise.

In his time, surgery has already separated largely from the rest of medicine and is far more active than in the Hippocratic writings. This evolution seems to have taken place particularly in Alexandria. We find indications for the following operations: polyps of the nose, glands of the neck, hernia, varicosity, suture of the large intestine, cutting of bladder stone. Catheters of bronze are employed. Other operations described are incision, the thread treatment of anal fisula, the couching of cataract, tonsillectomy. He gives excellent instructions for the treatment of fractures.

One of the most influential works of all medical history is the *Materia medica* of the Greek military surgeon Dioskorides, who served under Nero in the second half of the first century A.D. His influence goes far into modern times. Actually the German pharmacopoeia of 1910 still contained 90 drugs from Dioskorides. Dioskorides was a contemporary of Pliny, and both have apparently used a certain Kratoias, who lived in the first century B.C. Dioskorides describes altogether 950 curative substances, among them 600 plants (as compared to 250 of the Corpus Hippocraticum), 80 animals, and 50 minerals. In the introduction he recommends caution in collecting and storing the drugs, and uses smell and taste above all as criteria for the usefulness of a drug.

The work of Dioskorides is subdivided into five books. The first

deals with spices, oils, ointments, and trees. The second with animals, honey, milk, fat, cereals, and vegetables. The third with roots,
juices, herbs, and seeds. The fourth with the remaining herbs and
roots and the fifth with wines and metals.

We quote the following passage on iris, which is the first passage
in his book and which reflects very clearly the methods and concepts
of Dioskorides. He always describes according to a certain pattern,
which he repeats with all curative substances. First he discusses the
name and its synonyms. Then follows a botanical description, which
includes also a description of the subspecies. Then he enumerates
the curative virtues. Here he usually lacks very much a critical
attitude. For instance, iris cures such different afflictions as ulcers,
sleeplessness, bellyache, intoxications, spermatorrhea, irregularities of
menstruation, etc. Eventually he deals with the possibilities of preparing the drug.

Book One. Chapter 1. Iris. "Iris, the one call it the Illyric, others
thelpide, the heavenly, the cleaning, the miraculous, the Romans
marica, also gladiolus, opertritos, consecratix, the Egyptians Nar,
has its name on account of its similarity to the rainbow. Its leaves
resemble the sword lily, but they are larger and more brilliant. The
flowers are on stalks in equal distance, are reclined and colored
differently. One sees white, pale yellow, purple or bluish ones. On
account of the difference of the colors, it is compared to the rainbow
in the sky. The roots are subdivided, firm and smell good. They
are cut, dried in the shadow and are kept on a string. The best iris is
the Illyric and the Macedonian, and among those the most preferable
ones are those with many densely set, small roots, with mutilated
hard roots, which are of a pale yellow, smell well and burn the
tongue. The Lybian iris is not as strong, has a white color and a
bitter taste. When aging they are eaten by the worms, but the smell
improves and they have a warming strength and drive out, if put on
with twice as much white hellebore root, freckles and spots from sun-
burn. They fill ulcers with flesh, thin out excreta which are difficult to
throw out, and neutralize a poison when taken with fermented honey.
They produce sleep and tears, and cure bellyaches. Taken with
vinegar, they help those who have been bitten by poisonous animals,

also lienterics and those suffering from convulsions or from cold and chill and those suffering from spermatorrhea. Taken with wine they help menstruating, and a decoction is good for potency in women, because it softens and opens the passages. Introduced with honey, they drag out the embryo. Cooked in a cataplasm, they soften glands and old scars. They are also beneficial in headaches, if applied with vinegar and rose ointment. Eventually they are added to suppositories, plasters and ointments. They are useful in many conditions."

The second drug of Dioskorides, akoron, is a diuretic, helps in diseases of the chest and the liver, hernias, convulsions, women's diseases, eye diseases, intoxications, etc.

Dioskorides treats in the same manner in the first book Cyprus grass, calmus, bear root, Indian nard, Egyptian hazel root, Chinese cinnamon, Arab cassia, etc. It is interesting that among the first twenty-eight plants no less than twelve are "exotic," i.e., they are not Greek. They come from Egypt, India, China, and Arabia. Among the oils that now follow there is, of course, the unavoidable castor oil, and furthermore such strange things as the dirt from baths and gymnasia. Among the resins we find tar, asphalt, and naphtha. Among the trees laurel, plane-tree and poplar. Among the fruits acorns, dates, apples, and almonds.

Among the animals of the second book the most remarkable is the electric ray. The testicles of the hippopotamus are very warmly recommended just as are those of the beaver, which, for a long time, were used in the treatment of nervous conditions. Bugs are supposedly very helpful against quartan fever. Animal milk, fats (from goose to lion), blood, excrements, and urine are highly praised. Amongst the cereals and vegetables we find wheat, pumpkin, mustard, pepper, and scilla.

In the third book Dioskorides describes among other things gentian, sage, camomile, madder, and hemp. The fourth book contains above all narcotic solanaceas like mandragora, hyoscyamus, strychnine, atropa belladonna, datura stramonium and clematis, poppy, aconite, hemlock, helleborus and fern; altogether a fear-inspiring array of poisonous drugs. The fifth book deals with wines, mineral waters, and vinegar. Among metals zinc ointment is recommended very highly. Copper, iron, lead, and mercury are mentioned only as poisons. Used as medicaments are salts, coral, and other precious and semiprecious stones, arsenic, sulfur, and calcium.

The book of Dioskorides has always been praised very highly, especially by pharmacists. This is undoubtedly justified if we think only of the pharmaceutic aspect of Dioskorides. But from the therapeutic point of view we cannot overlook the fatal inclination of Dioskorides to make of every drug a panacea, which was not only quite naïve but certainly often detrimental to the patient and strengthened undoubtedly the tendency toward panaceas that appears again and again in the history of medicine.

In the early nineteenth century, Mérat pointed out the strange phenomenon that with the ancients, and even later, the same drug was simultaneously panacea and specific. Michler showed recently that humoral pathology, which disregards local therapy, automatically strengthens the tendencies toward panaceas. An idea that, by the way, then and later often paralyzed therapeutics is the idea of the largely hereditary nature of diseases.

Although it is perfectly legitimate to look at panaceas critically and negatively, it must be admitted that they are not exclusively the consequence of stupidity and laziness. They are the result of a conclusion by analogy which urgency and suffering of the sick in a way blackmail out of the physician: this drug has helped once, now it must also help in other cases. It is easy to observe the genesis of a panacea in a family, where the same substance that was so useful for mother in her abdominal troubles, now is taken by father against chest pain or by the son in states of exhaustion. The situation is often not so very different in the practice of the hard-pressed physician. The tragicomedy of the panacea is that substances, which without any doubt have very valuable specific effects, like digitalis, iodine, or quinine, are at times used against innumerable diseases against which nothing helps, but are no longer used for the disease in which they would really be curative.

This is possible because there is *one* panacea that in the most diverse diseases produces positive results: suggestion. Suggestion can improve the well-being of any patient, and suggestion can also produce in the physician illusions about the results he obtains.

V

Galen and Theriac

THE LAST great creative genius of Greek medicine, Galen of Perga-mon, A.D. 130–201, was primarily active in Rome, where he was the body physician of several emperors. Galen succeeded, at the end of the productive period of Greek medicine, in synthesizing various medical opinions, and for 1500 years this synthesis was dominant in Occidental medicine. It also contains a specific thera-peutic doctrine. It is no injustice to Galen to say that as an anatomist, physiologist, and pathologist he was far more eminent than as a therapist, although he boasts everywhere of his great therapeutic accomplishments. In view of his extraordinary influence, even Galen the therapist deserves our full attention.

Galen claims continuously to be the heir of Hippocrates. Actually he can be called a Hippocratist only in a very limited sense. In certain cases he did act as a Hippocratist, for instance in strongly emphasizing the importance of preventive hygienic measures, espe-cially in old people. Another example is his treatment of simple fevers, which consisted of bathing, massage, food diet, and evacua-tion. (His therapeutic procedures were directed primarily against fevers and inflammations.) Hippocratic, too, were his treatment of pulmonary tuberculosis with diet, fresh air, and roborants like arsenic, and his interest in the treatment of convalescents.

But in general the therapy of Galen is based far less on diet than that of the Hippocratists. And in his *Methodus medendi* he submits his diet ruthlessly to the four-quality pattern of humoral pathology: hot, dry, wet, cool. His prescriptions are primarily "wet" and "cool."

In bloodletting Galen, unlike the "vampires" of the seventeenth century, still considered age, sex, and state of the body as limita-tions, but he was considerably more inclined to bleed than the Hip-pocratists. He alternatively used enemas and bleeding.

Galen was far more liberal in the use of drugs than the Hippo-cratists. Max Neuburger once defined Galenism quite appropriately: "a combination of extensive drug treatment with the theoretical praise of nature as a healer."

The frequent use of bloodletting was excused with the patho-logical theory that disease is a plethora of bad humors. In blood-letting these humors were either derived ("derivatio," next to the focus, as it was practiced by the Hippocratists) or revolved ("revulsio," to a place distant from the focus, as it was practiced later on above all by the Arabs).

Galen made the use of drugs through his *Methodus medendi* more artificial and complicated than ever. Not only did he differentiate four qualities of disease causes and consequently four opposite qualities of drugs—this division is already very artificial, if we remember that, e.g., sea water is "dry" in it—but he subdivided each quality into no less than four degrees. The task of drugs was either to bring qualities into the body (metabole) or to change qualities in the body (alloiosis). According to Galen drugs had not only qualities but also so-called faculties, which in general are as meaningful as the famous saying of the candidate in the doctoral examination in the *Malade imaginaire* of Molière that opium has a soporific "faculty."

We must admit that Galen used these subdivisions in the attempt to individualize his therapeutics. Occasionally he tried to control his use of drugs, e.g., in self-experiments. Nevertheless one must say that the drug therapy of Galen was generally governed by a dull formalism proudly called "methodus" by him.

In general, Galen used drugs of plant origin without special chemical preparation. Therefore later on, in the period of chemiatry, such drugs were called galenics, as they were prescribed primarily by Galenists. The drugs of plant origin mentioned by Galen correspond more or less to those mentioned in Dioskorides. He was probably familiar with the book of Dioskorides.

Galen was particularly fond of that hellish brew called theriac. He discusses numerous theriac prescriptions. He always had to prepare the "theriac of Demetrios" for his emperor Marcus Aurelius, who by the way became an opium addict by taking this concoction. Through Galen and the Galenist Middle Ages, theriac became the great panacea.* The flesh of vipers in the theriac was regarded as

---

* In the third century B.C. two mixtures of herbs were used as antidotes. One of these mixtures was intended chiefly to prevent poisoning and was called mithridaticum in honor of the famous poisoner-king of Pontus. The other was primarily to invalidate animal poisons (those of snakes, spiders, etc.) and was later called theriac. Both mixtures were introduced into the prevention and treatment of infectious diseases, so-called pests. They remained always composed of herbs, but in the course of time minerals and animal parts were added. The poem of Nikander on theriac of 150 B.C. has become famous. Through the years a great many prescriptions for mithridaticum as well as theriac developed. The most famous prescription for theriac is that of

very important, just as hyoscyamus or the scilla mentioned previously in the *Papyrus Ebers*.

Galen also composed a list of so-called succedanea ("Ersatz"), which were supposed to help avoiding all too expensive drugs for patients with small income. He also described the numerous falsifications of drugs in his time. Smell and taste were to him again the main criteria in judging a drug. We find these criteria still in Barbier d'Amiens at the beginning of the nineteenth century!

It seems that Galen was originally, as far as medicaments are concerned, a skeptic. Even under the emperors such an attitude could be encountered occasionally. Galen's experiences with the public and his own temperament brought him soon on the road to poly-pharmacy and polypragmasy. It was his firm opinion that the public wants drugs (*populus remedia cupit*) and that expensive medicaments are more effective than cheap ones. He also promoted a strange theory that one should put into one preparation as many substances as possible. The body then would choose the ones that were useful to it. This is the theory of the so-called small-shot or shotgun pre-

---

Andromachos (a body physician to Nero), which also has been called galene. Andromachos introduced the use of the flesh of vipers in theriac. His theriac had 64 substances. There are prescriptions which have up to 100. These mixtures must have been very expensive.

It is reported that in the time of Galen rulers fearing poison took theriac prophylactically. Theriac became more and more a panacea. In the Middle Ages a true theriac industry developed in Italy, especially in Venice. From Venice it was exported as far as England, and during the great London plague of 1665 it was still consumed. For centuries there were complaints concerning peddlers who sold low-grade theriac as Venetian theriac. It is quite unlikely that theriac, either as an antidote or as a medicament, had any great effect. Nevertheless this expensive product was absorbed faithfully throughout centuries. With its incredible mixing, and the profound veneration devoted to its ineffectiveness, it is a symbol for a period of therapeutics which we dare hope belongs to the past. In the seventeenth century even a new theriac, called orvietan, caricatured by Molière, was invented.

Here too Enlightenment brought a change. Heberden published in 1745 his courageous little book against theriac. In 1788 theriac and mithridaticum disappeared from the London pharmacopoeia. In other places the evolution was much slower. In 1872 theriac was still found in the German pharmacopoeia, in 1884 in the French pharmacopoeia. When Claude Bernard around 1830 was an apothecary's apprentice in Lyon, he still had to prepare theriac. It is true, it was no longer done in solemn public ceremonies, as were customary in France, Germany, and Holland up to the end of the eighteenth century, in order to avoid falsifications. According to Claude Bernard all residues of medicaments were simply poured into a large vessel and this mixture was called theriac. *Sic transit gloria mundi!* It is not impossible that later generations will see some similarity between theriac and our own polypharmacy.

scriptions, of which the prototype was theriac and which have survived for a very long time.

The efforts of Galen to gain greater clarity in therapeutic procedures deserve commendation. He explained, e.g., that one should differentiate between the disturbed function and the pathological result of disturbed function, i.e., one should differentiate between symptom and cause. One should treat the latter, not the former. In discussing this matter he gives as example a case of treatment of limping in a phlegmone. He also tried to differentiate between drugs which change the body and food which only increases the substance of the body. In Galen we find the use of the medicament as a means of diagnosis "ex iuvantibus." If the substance, prescribed on the basis of a certain diagnosis, helps, the diagnosis was correct. This is a somewhat risky conclusion which nevertheless has been made again and again. We find relatively little magic in his writings, although magic had invaded therapeutics again considerably in his time. A large part of his therapeutic discussions, like all of his discussions, consists of rather unkind polemics with other physicians, especially with the schools of the methodists and empiricists. Galen also had a low opinion of surgery.

It is obvious that Galen had to be an enemy of the empiricists as well as the methodists. As much as he referred to Hippocrates and experience, he was as a therapist primarily a fanatic dogmatist. And whatever he claimed for his treatment, it was in reality overwhelmingly symptomatic.

How did Galen or a Galenist treat a disease so frequent and so dangerous in his time as pneumonia? We cite here the compilator, Paulus of Aegina, who depends entirely on Galen. If pneumonia is "primary," he prescribes venesection. In secondary, "converted" pneumonia one should give clysters and cup with scarification. Then one should give cathartic medicaments like bitter almonds, figs, and iris; one should anoint the thorax with irritating ointments and give plenty of liquid. This treatment is not essentially different from the Hippocratic one.

In comparison we now give the treatment of pneumonia by Soranus as it has been handed down to us in the book of Caelius Aurelianus on acute and chronic diseases.

Soranus of Ephesos, who lived around A.D. 100, was a member of the sect of methodists and was one of the most influential physicians of late antiquity; he was still known and respected in the early Middle Ages. The book of Caelius Aurelianus, which is only a Latin translation of the book of Soranus, is one of the most comprehensive and one of the few systematic medical books of antiquity.

In the case of pneumonia, Soranus suggests laying down the patient in a comfortable position, letting him fast for three days, and preventing him from sleeping through massage. This repulsive idea is explained by the fact that, according to the methodist doctrine, pneumonia is a status strictus which would get worse through sleep, which is strictus too. Furthermore Soranus recommends warm cataplasms.

After three days he gives warm water, allows sleep, and bleeds if the patient is strong enough. He now gives groats, sometimes only every second day. Then again warm cataplasms, cupping of the thorax and soft electuaries of pine kernels, fennel seeds, boiled honey, and egg yolk. Some of these medicaments are found in Hippocrates. Soranus also prescribes mild swinging, a kind of passive movement, as a therapeutic technique.

When the patient improves he gives more substantial food and wine, gives baths, and rubs the thorax with wax ointments and softening plasters.

As always in the book of Caelius Aurelianus–Soranus, we find polemics against the therapeutic indications of earlier physicians in connection with the positive suggestions of the author. For example, Soranus polemizes against the oxymel treatment of Hippocrates, the clysters of the dogmatic Diocles and his treatment with oxymel, aromatics, and other sharp medicaments. Soranus is also not in agreement with the famous Asklepiades, who opposed bloodletting and poultices, but he agrees with him in his refusal to give clysters in pneumonia. Passive movement, drinking of water, and pine kernels in the acute stage of the disease, as recommended by the methodist Themison, do not find his approval. The same holds for Themison's suggestion of cupping at the end of the disease. Furthermore Soranus opposes the numerous drugs of the empiricists. He mentions no less than seventeen prescribed by the sect.

We cannot find any essential difference or developments in the therapy of pneumonia up to the nineteenth century when skepticism, the antipyretic wave, eventually serums, and sulfanilamides changed the picture completely.

The long-lived therapeutic legacy of Galen, at least its tendency toward polypragmasy, polypharmacy, vampirism, and dogmatism and its negative attitude toward surgeons, cannot be evaluated very favorably. Neuburger writes not unjustly in his *Doctrine of the Healing Power of Nature*: "His epigones have even outdone Galen in therapeutic busybodyness. Thus it happened that in theory the principle that the physician is only the minister of nature was honored, but in reality, at the sick bed, an absolutely grotesque polypharmacy was practiced, and it was completely forgotten that sometimes it is a very good medicament not to use medicaments, as Hippocrates says in his *De articulationes*."

VI

Middle Ages

WITH GALEN, Greek medicine reaches the end of its creative period. It continues to exist as a fossil in Byzantium (Eastern Rome) in the work of Galenistic compilers such as Oribasius, Aetius, Alexander of Tralles, and Paulus of Aegina. In its own right, Byzantium makes a very original contribution in creating the first hospitals. In some Byzantine enclaves in the West, e.g., in Ravenna in the sixth century, Greek traditions are still alive. The therapeutics of this late Greek medicine are based on hygiene, polypharmacy, frequent bloodletting and "superstition," i.e., supernaturalistic ideas of a religious and magic, pagan and Christian nature.

In the monasteries of the West, the last refuges of Occidental scholarship, a medieval medicine, written in Latin, slowly grows; in general it is a rather shabby collection of translated Greek traditions mixed with Celtic and Germanic elements. Only through the Arabs did Greek traditions become accessible again on a large scale. Medical manuscripts from the fourth to the eleventh century are mainly collections of prescriptions, which are derived either from Galen or from Soranus. Through the Galen-worshipping Arabs the Soranus tradition is eventually eliminated in favor of the Galenic.

These collections of prescriptions are openly translations from the Greek, or they are so-called new creations in Latin, which are composed by North Africans like Vindicianus Afer and Theodorus Priscianus, or western European clerics like Marcellus Empiricus, Antimus, and Hrabanus Maurus. The official practitioners are again priests, a situation that offers the advantage that priests are able to treat without compensation, as they have income through their own profession. Their writings are either independent books or parts of encyclopedias. Some are entitled antidotaria, some receptaria. They are frequently anonymous.

We can visualize the therapeutics of this period not only through the collections of prescriptions, but also through the arrangement of the gardens of monasteries, which we find, e.g., in the history of the Benedictine monastery of Monte Cassino (founded in 528) as well as in the history of its descendants, the monasteries of St. Gallen and Schaffhouse, or in the *Hortulus* of the monk Walafried Strabo of the ninth century.

Walafried mentions in his poem, written about 825, concerning the garden of the monastery of Reichenau the following twenty-three plants and herbs: (1) sage (*Salvia officinalis*), (2) rue (*Ruta graveolens*) (3) lad's love (*Artemisia abrotanum*), (6) pumpkin (*Cucurbita lagenaria*), (5) melon (*Cucumis melo*), (6) vermouth (*Artemisia absinthum*), (7) hoarhound (*Marrubium vulgare*), (8) fennel (*Foeniculum vulgare*), (9) "gladiola" (a kind of iris), (10) lovage (*Levisticum officinale*), (11) chervil (*Scandix cerefolium*), (12) lily (*Lilium candidum*), (13) poppy (*Papaver*), (14) *Salvia sclarea*, (15) *Mentha piperita*, (16) *Mentha pulegium*, (17) celery (*Apium graveolens*), (18) *Betonica officinalis*, (19) agrimony (*Agrimonia eupatoria*), (20) "ambrosia," (21) hen-bit (*Nepeta cataria*), (22) radish (*Raphanus sativus*), and (23) rose.

Many of these plants appear also in the so-called Würzburg fever prescriptions, which Sticker published and which contain sixty-seven herbs (among them fifty-eight Greco-Roman ones), and in the instructions for gardening in the farms of Carolus Magnus (so-called capitularia) or in the map of the monastery of St. Gallen.

Far more extensive is the knowledge of healing herbs possessed by the abbess of Bingen, Hildegard (about 1150): forty-three planted in gardens, sixty-eight wild ones, and twenty-six imported plants (according to H. Fischer). During the thirteenth century the Salernitan, predominantly classic *Circa instans* of Matthaeus Platearius becomes the richest and most read herbal of western Europe.

Together with the medicaments and prescriptions of monastic medicine pagan superstition survived, partly translated into Christian ideas, as in the works of Hildegard of Bingen. Sleeping in the temple as a curative ritual was continued in Christian churches; and Christian saints, like Saint Cosmas or Saint Damian, specialized in miraculous cures. Almost none of these early medieval medical manuscripts deals with surgery and none with psychiatry or obstetrics.

Through contacts with the Arabs after the year 1000, partially established through the Crusades, western European Latin medieval medicine experiences a new impetus and takes on a new form While we have called the previous stage of medieval medicine the monastic, one could call this one the Arabistic or scholastic. During the seventh and eighth centuries the Arabs had, with the help of Byzantine and Jewish translators, in the newly conquered centers of the Near East like Bagdad and Damascus, assimilated the essential works of Greek medicine, organized them in their fashion, and made some additions. The very literary-minded Arabs became convinced Galenists. The therapeutic chapter in Avicenna's great teaching poem, e.g., starts with the Galenic slogan: "Contraria contrariis" (fight the opposite with the opposite, i.e., hot with cold, wet with dry, etc.), and a recommendation of purgatives to clean the humors.

The Arabs kept alive the Greek legacy concerning the necessity of hygiene and diet as therapeutic procedures far better than the early medieval Latin West, where the Roman baths and aqueducts had become ruins. The most famous Arab physician (the Arab physicians were not clerics like the scholastics of the West), the Persian Avicenna (980–1063), dealt a great deal with hygiene; several psychosomatic anecdotes concerning him are also reported. The great Jewish physician Moses Maimonides (1135–1205), who wrote in Arabic, was equally interested in psychosomatics and in hygiene. The other famous Persian-Arabic medical author, Rhazes (860–932), said in a truly Hippocratic spirit: "If you can cure with food, do not give drugs."

Rhazes gave a description of quacks which the eighteenth-century English medical historian Freind rightly said proved that numerous quacks were always at work and that they always proceeded in about the same fashion. Freind felt that the portrait of quacks as drawn by Rhazes was true to nature and that, had he lived in the eighteenth century, he would have found a considerable number of individuals resembling his picture.

We therefore quote here literally this famous passage from Rhazes: "Some pretend to cure epilepsy and make an opening at the occiput in the form of a cross and affirm to take out something which they kept in their hand before. Others make believe that they could extract snakes or lizards from the nose of their patients. In order to demonstrate this they put a pointed iron probe into a nostril and turn till blood comes. Then they extract a small artificial animal made from liver. Some claim that they could take the white spots out of the eyes. Before they insert the instrument, they put small pieces of cloth into the eye and then take them out with pincers and pretend to have extracted them directly from the eye. Still others assert that they could suck water out of the ear. To this effect they fill a tube from their mouth with water, hold the other end to the ear and then pretend that what in reality had come out of their mouth came out of the ear. Still others assert that they could remove worms which live in the ear or in the root of a tooth. Others bring out frogs from under the tongue which they have located there during the incision. What should I say about bones which are put into wounds and ulcers, and then extracted again after a certain lapse of time? Others state after an operation for bladder stone that there still remains one stone. They do this in order to make believe that they have extracted at least one. Others probe the bladder, although they have no idea whether there is a stone or not. But if they do not find one, they pretend to have extracted at least one, which they keep ready and show to this effect. Sometimes they make an incision at the anus for hemorrhoids and thus produce a fistula or an ulcer, which did not exist before. Some claim to remove phlegm from the penis or other parts of the body by way of a pipe which they hold filled in their mouth. Some pretend that they could concentrate all humors of the body in one single place by rubbing it with winter cherries. This produces a burning or a slight inflammation. Then they want to be paid as if they had cured the disease. When they then put oil on this inflamed part, the pain actually disappears.

"Some convince their patients that they have swallowed some glass and by introducing a feather into their throat they make them vomit what they have introduced with that same feather. Many objects come out of the body which the crooks have inserted with great dexterity and therewith endangered the health of their patients and even brought about their death. Such swindle should not be possible with critical people, but these do not dream of such frauds and do not doubt the skill of those who use it. The deception is only discovered when they get suspicious and look more closely at these operations. Therefore no intelligent person should put his life into the hands of quacks or take of their drugs, which have killed so many."

It is regrettable that the Arabs practiced polypharmacy even more than Galen. They were able to do so because accessible to these indefatigable travelers and conquerors were not only the whole Greek pharmacopoeia—they were eager students of Dioskorides— but also the whole pharmacopoeia of India. This is clearly visible from the work of their greatest pharmacologist and botanist, Ibn al Baitar (died in 1248), who knew no less than 2000 substances, of which 145 were from the mineral kingdom, 130 from the animal kingdom, the rest from the vegetable kingdom. Ibn al Baitar grew up in the other great center of Arabic culture, in Spain, but returned to Syria at the end of his life.

The Arabs were probably the first to introduce chemically prepared mineral substances on a large scale into therapeutics, especially mercury, which was then used and abused for such a long time. Calomel was later called "panacea mineralis." The western European Arabists took over mercury from the Arabs. It was no accident that the Arabs were the first to use these chemically prepared substances, as they were very much attracted by alchemy, an early form of chemistry.

Rhazes himself was a well-known alchemist and performed experiments with chemical substances. In spite of these attempts to proceed empirically, the Arabs also adopted faithfully such supposed "results of experience" of the past as the claim that the flesh of vipers or castration can cure leprosy.

Superstitious and pseudoscientific elements play a great role in Arabic medicine. We have mentioned the pseudoscience alchemy, which contains elements of a future chemistry, but as a whole is a mystic, secret search for the transmutation of metals, the stone of wisdom, the quintessence, the elixir of life, etc. In connection with such ideas we better understand the high respect for the therapeutic value of ground precious stones which was held by the Arabs and their later imitators in the West. Alchemical ideas like that of the stone of wisdom are based simultaneously on the faith in panaceas.

Astrology too played a major role in Arabic practice, although leading Arab physicians like Avicenna, Avenzoar, and Averroes were no friends of this superstition.

It is interesting that the Arabs frequently prepared arsenic ointments. Since the time of the Arabs the use of arsenic resembles that of a panacea. The Arabs greatly increased the number of prescriptions for counterpoisons (Alexipharmaka), which they also used to treat those diseases that we know today to be infections, yet which they regarded as poisoning.

It was undoubtedly of great importance for the whole further development of therapeutics that the Arabs, probably in Bagdad as early as the last quarter of the eighth century, developed independent apothecary shops, in the beginning probably in connection with hospitals.

Besides the use of hygiene and of numerous drugs the Arabs had an inclination toward venesection, as we can see without difficulty from the writings of Rhazes and Avicenna. They surrounded venesection with complicated theoretical discussions (revulsion or derivation).

With the exception of Abul Kasim of Cordoba (died 1013) the Arabs had little interest in surgery. Avicenna thought surgery to be something of low value. The same holds true for obstetrics. They excelled only in one single type of operation: eye operations. Their predilection for the hot iron as a means of stopping bleeding unfortunately also diffused in the West and formed a serious impediment for the further evolution of surgery.

Arabic medicine conquered the West via southern Italy, Spain, and southern France. The main artisans of this conquest were the authors who translated Arabic materials into Latin, like Constantinus Africanus (1020–1087), who worked in Salerno and in the monastery Monte Cassino, and Gerard of Cremona (1140–1187), who lived in Toledo. The first Arabistic school of the Christian West was Salerno which experienced its greatest flowering in the twelfth century. The representative Salernitan antidotarium Nicolai is full of Arab drugs like castor oil, camphor, bezoar, musk, senna, nux vomica, hemp, and mercury. In Salerno the ashes of sponges containing iodine were used against goiter. Hygienic rules were contained in the so-called Regimen Salernitanum, which probably did not originate in Salerno, but which shows through its name that Salerno was regarded as the source of hygienic teaching. Some of the rules of this regimen, famous for so many centuries, survive today in popular tradition. From Salerno some remarkable surgical accomplishments are reported, such as suture of the intestine. Unfortunately here, too, the Arab hot iron eventually dominated the scene.

In order to gain a concrete idea of the accomplishments of therapeutics in the Middle Ages, it is perhaps best if we study the report of the treatment of the Byzantine emperor Alexis in 1118, as his daughter Anna has transmitted it to us. The emperor suffered since 1107, i.e., since his sixtieth year, from periodic painful swellings of

his feet, which in true Galenist fashion were designated as "rheumatism." In 1118 the same affliction appeared in the shoulders. Some
physicians recommended purgatives; the majority opposed. As the
emperor kept a rigid diet, no dietary fault could be diagnosed.
Thus he supposedly suffered from inflammation of the heart, resulting
from the worries of governing. In the framework of Galenism it is
rather surprising that a disease of the heart was diagnosed. The
emperor suffered more and more from shortness of breath. He was
no longer able to lay down. Venesections did not accomplish anything. An antidote from pepper brought relief only for four days.
Change of climate did not help either. Now the abdomen began to
swell and fever appeared. The emperor was then cauterized, but
without success, and he died within eleven days.

The therapeutics of the legendary Arnald of Villanova (1235–
1312)—a court physician in different places of the Mediterranean
area, who had studied and taught in Montpellier—seem very typical
for the therapeutics of full-blown medical scholasticism. For Arnald,
a Christian, the basis of medicine is not only Galenic reason and
experience, but Christian revelation. Basically, as with almost all
medieval authors, authority of the past is the essential thing. This
becomes obvious when we observe his numerous Avicenna quota-
tions, or his imitation of the humoral theories with their qualities
and secondary qualities, and especially when we learn from him
that dosage of a substance has to be decided according to the majority opinion of ancient authors.

According to Paul Diepgen, Arnald had anti-Galenist traits. I
must confess that I have not succeeded in finding them. It is true
that he defends such points of view, which appear reasonable to us,
as the opposition against composed drugs and shows much understanding for the necessity of good care in convalescence; and we
find such sentences as "use rather food than drugs." But this can
also be found in Galen. Therefore Arnald's "anti-Galenist" manifes-
tations of reason remained probably rather theoretical.

In reality Arnald is an enthusiastic partisan of theriac, the opiates,
and gold (he, too, was a famous alchemist), which is supposedly
particularly good in heart disease. He is a fervent admirer of cathartics, just like his contemporary Gilbertus Anglicus. Gilbertus
wanted once to reduce the use of drugs to a minimum, but he found

that patients do not like this. Besides cathartics, Arnald recommends the so-called metasyncritic treatment. This is one of the few traces of methodist opinions to be found in his writings. Besides cathartics Arnald recommends, like many of his contemporaries, cupping.

Eventually Arnald is a great friend of venesection. Venesections in the Middle Ages were of a rather energetic kind. The patient lost from 100 to 1000 grams. Galen connected bloodletting with the phases of the moon. Arnald and his contemporaries not only followed him in this, but connected in general very closely astrology and bloodletting.

It is interesting to notice that Arnald recommends the use of passions and the mobilization of imagination in order to further the healing process. On the physical side of medicine he insists on examination of drinking water for hygienic safety. Arnald, too, was an alchemist and believed in the quinta essentia of Raimundus Lullus, who supposedly had been his disciple in alchemy.

That bloodletting plays a tremendous role in scholastic medicine is also evident from the writings of Pietro d'Abano (1250–1320), which also contain numerous magic elements, and from the writings of the papal court surgeon Guy de Chauliac and of Albertus Magnus. A further indication of the prevalence of bloodletting is the "bloodletting men" who are found in the early medical prints of the late Middle Ages and in Ketham. As a measure of prevention, monks were bled several times during a year by the monastery barber. Medieval bloodletting was practiced in general the Arabic way, i.e., as revulsio (on the side of the body opposed to the diseased side).

Galenist medieval physicians, e.g., Vincent de Beauvais, still paid lip service to hygiene. But these writings do not give the impression that they are based on actual hygienic activities, but rather impress as mechanical imitations of antiquity. For one hygienic activity we possess numerous later medieval treatises: bathing. Giacomo de Dondis (born in 1298), professor in Padua, studied, e.g., the salts of mineral waters.

The many plague treatises of the late Middle Ages—from 1347 into the eighteenth century, bubonic plague was endemic in Europe —reveal a tremendous helplessness. It is not surprising that the antischolastic Petrarca mocked contemporary medicine. He regarded dietetics and surgery as its only positive features.

Very important therapeutic contributions of the Middle Ages were the invention of eyeglasses in the thirteenth century and the foundation of numerous hospitals.

In western Europe the Arab example was imitated in the decisive step of separating pharmacy from medicine. This is laid down in the famous southern Italian health laws of 1240 edicted by the king of Sicily and German emperor Frederic II, which created fee schedules for apothecary products and assigned apothecaries to certain guilds. Later such laws are increasingly found all over Europe.

The compendium of Saladin of Ascolo, written in 1488, is the first true book for apothecaries. He intended, as he says, to improve with this book the very defective knowledge of the aromatarii (apothecaries). The first official pharmacopoeia dates from 1498 and originated in Florence. The fact that a profession of apothecary developed in the cities, and that the number of pharmacists grew, shows that the number of city dwellers and townsmen, as well as the use of drugs, increased during the Middle Ages. On the other hand, it is obvious that the existence of pharmacies was a stimulus for drug treatment.

Surgery in the Middle Ages was not very developed. The physicians had abandoned surgery as early as the end of antiquity, and surgery was practiced in the Middle Ages mostly by craftsmen who worked simultaneously as barbers or bathkeepers. Nevertheless medieval surgery shows some fine accomplishments. The surgical writings of the Salernitan school show a certain competence. In Bologna under Hug, Theodoric, and Saliceto there developed a certain surgical tradition which Lanfranco brought to France and which was brilliantly represented there by Henri de Mondeville and Guy de Chauliac. The Arabist influence was very unfavorable for surgery, as the Arabs thought little of it, and they preferred the hot iron to the knife. Bertapaglia furthermore points to the fact that surgeons used too many drugs.

Insofar as the Middle Ages did possess a scientific therapy, it was dominated by the unholy trinity of Galen: venesection, evacuation, drugs. While the Greco-Roman elements of the pharmacopoeia shrunk, pharmacopoeias were enlarged through native drugs, drugs coming from the East, and chemical drugs, which were applied poorly. The great mass of the population were therapeutically left more or less to themselves, to some old men and women and the saints. It is typical that, in order to remedy the situation, special collections of cheap prescriptions for poor people were created, such as the *Thesaurus pauperum* of Petrus Hispanus (middle of the thirteenth century). This custom had begun in antiquity with Ammonius Serenus and continued up into the nineteenth century; in 1812 Hufeland published an *Armenapotheke* (poor men's pharmacy).

In the framework of this book we can unfortunately give only the European therapeutic tradition. We would nevertheless like to mention briefly the medicine of two Eastern cultures which have at least reached the level of European antiquity and of medieval medicine and which have enriched Western medicine again and again by isolated therapeutic elements: India and China.

It is difficult to date Indian medicine. Estimates concerning the writing of its great classics, e.g., Susruta, oscillate between 900 B.C. and A.D. 800. The basic ideas of Indian medicine are those of a speculative humoral pathology. They are mixed with many supernaturalistic elements and pseudosciences like astrology. They seem to date from the eighth to the fourth century B.C. In Indian medicine diet is extremely important, and it is interesting to note that the Indian classics prescribe a salt-free diet in dropsy. With the Hindus we find a respect for diet similar to that of the Greeks. We also encounter numerous drugs. An Indian drug, rauwolfia, described by Garcia da Orta in 1563, opened up, one and a half decades ago, as reserpine a new epoch in psychiatric therapeutics, the so-called psychopharmaceuticals.

Susruta describes, besides mineral and animal medicaments, 600 plants. He subdivides medicaments according to the diseases in which they are supposed to be helpful. Cathartics, emetics, and bloodletting are recommended frequently. It is known to him that abuse of these therapeutic procedures can bring about diseases, and these diseases are described.

Indian surgery, which knew amputation, protheses, and plastic operations, was brilliant. Susruta describes no less than 125 instruments. Psychic cause of disease and psychological treatment were well known to the Hindu medical classics. There is no doubt that Hindu medicine very strongly influenced the Greeks as well as the Chinese.

Chinese medicine too is very old and equally hard to date. Dating its classics at 2900 B.C. is probably a fancy. Its medicine is based on a five-element doctrine, and these five elements are related to five planets, five seasons, five colors, five sounds, five directions, and five organs.

The Chinese, who also had apothecary shops, had developed drug lore to a very high level. They knew no less than 1800 drugs. The drug Ma Huang (*Ephedra vulgaris*) was used by them for 4000 years in weak circulation, treatment of fever, coughing, and as a stimulant for slaves. In 1887 ephedrine was isolated by Nagai and in 1924 introduced in the West by the Chinese-American pharmacologist Chen. Other Chinese drugs, which in recent times have played a certain role in Western medicine, are chaulmoogra oil and buffagine. Rhubarb and camphor have been known to the Chinese for a very long time. They regarded camphor as a panacea, and via the Arabs the West inherited this error. Other panaceas of theirs were gold powder and ginseng. The Chinese have used for a long time cod liver oil and *Secale cornutum* (ergot), also iron, arsenic, and mercury preparations as well as calcium in the form of the so-called dragon bones (which in reality are fossilized bones). Arsenic was used by them in conditions that were probably caused by syphilis. Although the Chinese were very strongly influenced by the Hindus in medical matters, they did not accept bloodletting or surgery, which did not correspond to their basic orientation. On the other hand, they developed particularly massage, cupping, and gymnastics. Two therapeutic techniques used as panaceas, acupuncture and moxa, have for about 300 years now been periodically introduced into Western medicines. In the first years after their introduction very good successes were reported. Then silence surrounded these techniques till they were rediscovered, usually when China became fashionable for cultural or political reasons.

VII

Renaissance

THE RENAISSANCE in medicine, which occurs in the sixteenth century, is very important in the history of therapeutics. The majority of the official curers are again laymen, nonpriests. The upper strata of society are now taken care of by the academic group of physicians, which had developed during the Middle Ages. The majority of the population is at best taken care of by barber-surgeons, bathkeepers, traveling doctors, apothecaries, but is also not rarely in the hands of hangmen and untrained practitioners of all kinds.

During this period the decomposition of ancient tradition begins, which will lead into an increasing therapeutic chaos. This chaos will reach its acme in the nineteenth century, and then change into a new and incomparably more effective therapy. It seems reasonable to regard the numerous medical "systems" of the following two centuries as an attempt to overcome this chaos. During the Renaissance many valuable old medical data were revived. And extremely important new tendencies became effective for the first time on a large scale. New experiences were registered.

At the beginning of the medical Renaissance the most important thing for therapists was medical herb lore. This conclusion is imperative if we note that the oldest printed medical books, so-called incunabula, i.e., those printed before 1500, are herbals. Equally typical is the enthusiasm for Dioskorides which manifests itself in many translations and new editions, of which the best known is that by Mattioli.

Of the three most famous innovators of the medical Renaissance, Vesal contributed next to nothing to a renovation of therapeutics. He corrected Galen's erroneous anatomy, but he remained a humoral pathologist, and his reviving, or more exactly new creation, of anatomy was not immediately applicable in therapeutics, except for surgery. But the two other pillars of Renaissance medicine—Paracelsus and Paré—have influenced therapeutics very strongly in a sense of renovation.

Paracelsus brought a second great turning point into the history of therapeutics, not inferior in importance to the turning point brought about by the Greeks through secularization of therapeutics after the seventh century B.C. Paracelsus was born in 1493 in Einsiedeln, Switzerland. His father was a descendant of a Swabian noble family, von Hohenheim. Paracelsus' original name was Theophrast of Hohenheim. He started a change in medicine that, in content and in language, deserves to be called a revolution. Paracelsus was the first to refuse the Galenic theory of humors, which had been the basis of all therapeutics for most ancient authors and for nearly all of the Middle Ages. Paracelsus, alchemist and metallurgist, dethroned drugs of plant origin, which had been dominant so far. He abandoned the Greek principle of treating the state of the patient in favor of specific treatment. This specific treatment is with him a kind of secularized, chemical exorcism. Specific treatment in a scientific form has, after Paracelsus, come more and more to the foreground. Paracelsus and his partisans, the so-called spagyrics, who were chemists, started a 100-year-long war with the orthodox Galenists, who used only natural, not chemically changed products. This battle ended with the victory of the spagyrics. Later on, not only many eclectics but even many physicians with Galenist sympathies used spagyric preparations, as we will see in the next chapter.

Paracelsus was an alchemist. For him alchemy was one of the four columns of medicine. The other three were nature, god, and astrology. The alchemy of Paracelsus is, like his whole thinking, a strange mixture of empiricism and speculation. As an alchemist he owed, of course, much to the Arabs. As a true demagogue he violently cursed the Arabs while, however, using their discoveries. The same holds true for his attitude toward Galen. Sticker has demonstrated that many of his ideas, like the one that nature "eliminates" disease, show a clear relationship with Galenic ideas.

The physiology of Paracelsus was alchemistically colored. The body was governed by the so-called archeus, a master alchemist, who had his seat in the region of the stomach. When disease generated, such alchemistic processes as transmutations of diseases or transplantations of natural bodies took place in the organs, which resembled very much alchemist kitchens. The principle of Paracelsus was: for new chemical diseases (the fact that there are new diseases was explained by astrology), new chemical remedies and a new physician are needed. Paracelsus was particularly hostile against apothecaries and against the use of guaiac wood.

The notion of specifics—i.e., the driving out of certain disease entities through certain medicaments—is derived in large part from Paracelsus. But such a notion must somehow have already been in the air. It is, e.g., also found in the great contemporary of Paracelsus, who otherwise resembled him so little, Fracastorius. The notion of specifics implies that now the disease, and no longer the diseased and his state, is treated. It is therefore not surprising that Paracelsus practically never mentions diet. He called his specifics arcana, i.e., secret remedies. These arcana were chemically prepared as extracts or tinctures, which contain the quintessence of the substances. Paracelsus knew seven ways to find specifics.

In plant specifics—Paracelsus did use plants, too—he adhered to the doctrine of the so-called signatures. Signatures are a magic notion. According to the doctrine of signatures, form and color of an object announce its therapeutic destination: leaves in the form of kidneys are good against kidney diseases, yellow flowers against jaundice, etc. This idea is found in primitive medicine, too.

As an alchemist Paracelsus used above all minerals. Mercury, e.g., plays a tremendous role in his treatment of syphilis. He used it more reasonably than many of his contemporaries, or even later physicians like Sydenham, who made his poor syphilitics produce, by means of mercury poisoning, four quarts of saliva per day. Paracelsus was also the first to use mercury as a diuretic.

Other minerals used by Paracelsus were arsenic and its compounds, which were now given more and more orally, sulfur, lead, copper, iron, silver, gold, and antimony.

Antimony was the favorite of Paracelsus and his disciples. It was given not only in several compounds but also in the strange form of pilulae eternae, which were fished out of the excrement again and again, cleaned and taken anew. From Paracelsus to Rasori antimony functioned as a panacea and was often called panacea antimonica. The most widespread antimony preparation was tartar emetic. Antimony was, during the sixteenth and seventeenth centuries, the main bone of contention between Galenists and Paracelsists. Here they separated. A physician who prescribed antimony was no reliable anti-Paracelsist. In 1566 the Galenists obtained in their capital Paris the interdiction of antimony. In 1666 the spagyrics triumphed when the interdiction was revoked.

Paracelsus was very much interested in bathing, not so much because of the physical effects of baths, but on account of the content in minerals in different sources, which he examined. Paracelsus used in addition many mysterious medicaments like mummy, scraped skull, precious stones (these are found even in such a sober therapist as Felix Platter), and unicorn. He also prescribed amulets, and Walter Pagel seems absolutely correct in regarding him rather as a "magus" than as a modern scientist. Paracelsus did not abandon old-fashioned plant drugs like helleborus, camphor, lilium convallaria, and mint-balm.

He is supposed to have been a good surgeon. As he was a partisan of sympathetic (i.e., magic) powders, which were applied not to the wound but to the weapon that had produced the wound, his wounds probably really closed much better than those that had been treated with the whole ointment junk of the apothecaries of his time. If one wishes, one can regard Paracelsus as a kind of involuntary psychotherapist. His proposition to curse waxen images of enemies in psychological difficulties had undoubtedly positive psychological effects. Paracelsus belongs to that group of Renaissance physicians who saw that so-called imaginatio, a psychological phenomenon which we call today suggestion, could create as well as cure disease.

For a while Paracelsus divided diseases simply according to the remedies that supposedly cured them. Thus he constructed a morbus helleboricus, a morbus terpentinus, etc. This strange attempt was repeated in the nineteenth century by Rademacher. Paracelsus talked a lot about the healing force of nature, but actually he was, following his temperament and his conviction, a very active therapist. He believed firmly that there did exist a drug against every disease. This was not the only contradiction in his therapeutic doctrine. In his book *On the French Disease* (i.e., syphilis), he claims that the remedies for German diseases must be found in Germany: "How can the remedy for the Rhine grow at the Nile?" In his *Tartaric Diseases*, he says exactly the contrary, i.e., that remedies are found in foreign countries. In the last instance Paracelsus believes that the cure is accomplished by God, not by nature. Also in many other respects Paracelsus is very contradictory in his therapeutics. He preaches individualization, but always looks for a universal medicine. He preaches simplification of prescriptions, but writes himself extremely long prescriptions. He condemns bloodletting, only to recommend it warmly in other places. He is the protagonist of specifics, but he also invented a panacea. As an alchemist he knows the experiment well, but as a mystic "experientia" is to him more than just prosaic experiment. To him it is a mystic union with the object, something closely related to religious experience.

Very typical for Paracelsus are his *Nine Books about Chemistry and the Cure of the French Disease,* published in 1528. This is one of the few works of Paracelsus published during his lifetime. The first thirteen chapters consist almost exclusively of the crudest invectives against all those who in his time treated the French disease. He calls them cheats, crooks, hangmen, etc. Even the later chapters abound with such "polite" statements. He very energetically opposes the use of mercury and its abuse, but his prescriptions that follow contain a great many mercury preparations. He declares in the very same chapter abstention from food as being something unnecessary as well as being something very useful. In spite of all these strange facts, the role of Paracelsus and his disciples for the further evolution of therapeutics in the direction of chemical remedies and specifics has been an extremely important one.

The second new and decisive element in the therapeutics of the Renaissance was the introduction of exotic drugs which had a great practical and theoretical effect. They undermined ancient tradition in no less an effective way than the curses of Paracelsus. It now became obvious that the book of Dioskorides contained by no means the total drug lore of the world and that neither the Greeks nor the Arabs possessed absolute truths in this domain.

The new drugs the Europeans found in America (the "West Indies") were described primarily by Hernandez, Monardes, and Acosta. The most important descriptions of the drugs of those countries that now became far better known through new sea routes, the "East Indies," i.e., India and Indonesia, are found in the works of Garcia da Orta and Rauwolf. Guilandinus, Prosper Alpino, and Belon studied the herbs in less distant regions like the Balkans and Egypt. Clusius wrote the first large compendium of the newly discovered drugs.

The opportunity to acquire spices and drugs through trans-Atlantic expansion served as a very important stimulus for movements that were to have grave economic and political consequences.

The following drugs were introduced from America: guaiac, recommended by Hutten as well as Fernel as an antisyphilitic; sarsaparilla (also an antisyphilitic); Peru balm; tolubalm; lobelia; cascara sagrada; chenopodium; cocaine; curare; and tobacco. The last-named was used in the beginning primarily as a drug with a clear tendency toward a panacea. The so-called tobacco clyster lasted from John Woodall (born 1569) to Sir Benjamin Brodie (1783–1862). The two most important American drugs, ipecacuanha and cinchona, reached Europe pharmacopoeias only in the seventeenth century.

Europeans were overwhelmed by the knowledge of plants possessed by American Indians. Hernandez, the body physician of the Spanish king, was sent by the latter to study American medicinal herbs and reported that the Mexicans knew no less than 3000 plants. Europeans acquired from the natives of the Americas not only medicinal plants but also plant food like potatoes and stimulants like maté and cacao.

Not only exotic drugs were searched for. In the course of the revival of botany, European drugs were studied too. It was necessary to have healing herbs for the common man. The exotic drugs were far too expensive for him. Intensive study of the flora of their own country brought with it the discovery of numerous new species and a thorough criticism of the writings of Dioskorides and Pliny. This critical revival of botany was of the utmost importance for medicine, as its therapeutic armamentarium still consisted primarily of plants. The new botany was almost exclusively the work of physicians. We mention among the great reformers of botany only Mattioli, Amatus Lusitanus, Cesalpino, Leonicenus, Ruelle, Belon, Conrad Gessner (who also studied chemical remedies and is one of the first physicians who reports therapeutic self-experiments), Brunfels, Bock, Valerius Cordus, and Fuchs. The last, who is very representative for his time, knows 488 species of healing plants as compared to 243 of the Hippocratists and 600 of Dioskorides.

During the sixteenth century the first German pharmacopoeias were written, the Nürnberg one by the botanist Valerius Cordus in 1546, the Augsburg one by Occo in 1564, the Cologne one by Faber and others in 1565, etc.

Thus during the sixteenth century a firm, centuries-old therapeutic structure was shaken in its foundations and a chaos that was to last four hundred years began. This becomes particularly visible if we

study the problem of bloodletting. Up to this time very few differences
of opinion concerning bloodletting had arisen. Now the controversy
around the Parisian Pierre Brissot rose. Brissot wanted to return
from Arabist revulsion to ancient derivation. Brissot was regaded as
a worse heretic than Luther and died in 1522 in Portuguese exile.

Some now questioned bloodletting altogether. Krato von Kraftheim
as well as Fracastorius were so-called hematophobes and were very
hesitant when it came to bleeding. This attitude is connected with a
return to observation, to conservative, expectative practice, and confidence in the healing power of nature, as symbolized by Hippocrates.
This attitude was represented during the medical Renaissance by
Baillou, Valleriola, Cesalpino, Johannes Lange, and others. The more
frequent expectative attitude, and the use of natural methods like
gymnastics (Mercurialis, Santorio), baths (Rivière), etc., was perhaps more useful to the patients of that period than all spagyrics
and discoverers of America taken together.

Others propagated a very intensive therapeutic activity, especially
in the field of bloodletting. We have already mentioned Paracelsus.
Much worse were Mercurialis (his battle cry was: bleeding, bleeding,
bleeding) and Botallus (born in 1530). These tendencies were
continued during the seventeenth century by Riolan and Guy Patin.
They explain perhaps the observation of Santorio that during a
plague epidemic the rich people, who were treated, died, while the
poor, who were not treated, survived.

A similar activistic misuse began in the field of mercury treatment, which increased automatically with the spread of the diagnosis
syphilis during the sixteenth century. Fernelius, Fallopius, Montanus,
Vidius, and Lange voiced in vain their warnings against this toxic
habit. In spite of further protestations it was continued throughout
the following centuries. The therapy of syphilis offered an opportunity to try all existing remedies in the worst extreme form, in
general without any profit, but with lots of damage. The cruelty of
these therapeutics was often conscious and an intended punishment
to the sinner. We remind only of the flogging and fasting before
drugs were given. J. K. Proksch reports no less than 2000 drugs
that were used in the course of time against syphilis. During the
seventeenth century even trepanation was introduced. On the other

hand, many so-called antimercurialists declared many symptoms of syphilis to be symptoms of mercury poisoning.

Clysters seem to have increased during the sixteenth century. It is probably no accident that Paré, who was a natural inventor—he invented also the mechanical sacrificator, artificial limbs, orthopedic apparatus, etc.—created the self-clystering syringe.

The barber-surgeon Ambroise Paré (1510–1590) from Laval is a leading figure in the Renaissance of surgery. His most important accomplishments are the reintroduction of the ligature to stop bleeding, the improvement of the abominable treatment of wounds produced by gunpowder weapons (a reform that was also preached by the Italian Maggi), and the reintroduction of podalic version of the feet in obstetrics. The contributions of Paré are not limited to surgery. Very important for therapeutics was his attack on the fashionable drugs mummy and unicorn, which, in addition, were very expensive. The unicorn is one of the most interesting animals in medical history. It never existed, yet its horn was extremely expensive and was used everywhere, especially as counterpoison, as antidote. In reality it seems that the teeth of the narwhal were sold as unicorns' horns.

Paré is by no means the only important surgeon of the sixteenth century. At least as important were contemporaries like Pierre Franco, a Provençal Huguenot, who lived most of his life in Switzerland and who considerably improved the traditional quack operations: cutting the stone, operating on cataract and hernias. Or Tagliacozzi, the first scientific physician in Europe who practiced plastic surgery. Jakob Ruff, Felix Würtz, Brunschwig, etc., deserve mention too. In view of the fact that the surgeons remained up into the nineteenth century the healers of the large masses of the population, their level of practice is very important for the general therapeutic picture.

During the sixteenth century no theory of experience exists. But experience itself enters therapeutics with the treatment of the wounds produced by the new firearms, with the treatment of the "new" syphilis—both mainly undertaken by surgeons—and with the importation of exotic drugs. It is typical that Ambroise Paré reports a clinical experiment with controls in treating burns and Conrad Gessner his self-experiments with nicotine.

VIII

Therapeutics in the
Seventeenth Century

THE MAIN tendencies in therapeutics during the sixteenth century, i.e., during the Renaissance, are Galenist traditionalism, the chemiatrics of Paracelsus and his disciples, the new botany, the importation of exotic drugs, and the revival of "Hippocratism." All these tendencies continue during the seventeenth century. Added are iatrophysics and skepticism.

One can practice Galenist traditionalism—which therapeutically means, above all, evacuation, especially by venesection, contraria contrariis, and drugs from the vegetable kingdom—in a relatively reasonable fashion as it was done, e.g., by P. Pigray (1532–1613), M. Lister (1638–1711), or Richard Morton (1637–1698). The latter does not hesitate, in spite of his traditionalism, to add to his armamentarium chemiatric or other drugs that seem useful to him, like the cortex peruviana (our quinine).

Traditionalism can be, on the other hand, extremely narrow-minded, schematic, and deadly, as in the hands of the notorious Paris dean Guy Patin (1601–1672) and his followers. With them bloodletting and purging became very dangerous panaceas. Patin wrote in 1652: "All diseases can be cured with the syringe, the lancet, cassia, senna, and syrup of roses and peach flowers." He was a deadly enemy of the apothecaries, because they sold antimony. He bled, e.g., a seven-year-old boy with pleurisy thirteen times in two weeks, his own three-year-old grandson twice in bronchitis. During the same time he bled his son for tuberculosis twenty times, himself for a toothache twice and for a "bilious" disease six times. In addition, of course, he purged. He almost never reports a death of patients. This is no proof that it did not occur. He was by no means the only therapist of this kind. He tells triumphantly that his colleague, the body physician Cousinot, was bled by his father and father-in-law, both physicians, for rheumatism 64 times in eight months and then purged thoroughly. Poor King Louis XIII was during one year bled 47 times, received 212 clysters, and 215 purges. It is hard to tell which form of traditionalism was prevalent—the one practiced by Morton or the one practiced by Patin. Probably it was the latter, which was continued by Chirac and others into the next century. The descriptions of Molière of these healing artists have been regarded as exaggerations. They might be understatements. Next to clysters bathing in spas was very fashionable during this century. It was a strange mixture of hygienic therapeutic measures and mundane happenings. The same holds true for later times.

The great opponents of traditionalism and probably the most important current in therapeutics during the seventeenth century were the chemiatrists, the followers of Paracelsus, who refused blood-letting and were therefore so vehemently cursed by Patin. On account of their declination to bleed, J. G. Zimmermann called them later contemptuously "mere apothecaries." The influence of the chemiatrists during the seventeenth century is no accident. During this century several thousand books on alchemy were published and the Rosicrucian order was very strong.

The chemiatrists introduced numerous chemically prepared drugs, often of mineral origin. Antimony, the "regulus" of the alchemists, condemned by the Parisian faculty and parliament in 1566, rehabilitated in 1666, was, as mentioned previously, the main bone of contention between traditionalists and chemiatrists. This makes it for the historian a "guiding fossil." Although once in a long time a Galenist (e.g., Masaria) might prescribe antimony, in general one can assume that an author who prescribes antimony is no enemy of the chemiatrists. With the help of the Paracelsists calomel, used so much in later times, began its career around 1600. Chemical drugs of mineral origin had one aspect that was very attractive for many physicians. They could be quantified. Three grams of calomel were pharmacologically always identical with three grams of calomel, while three grams of Peruvian cortex or three grams of root of ipecacuanha were not identical on account of the great fluctuations in alkaloid content in natural drugs.

During the seventeenth century chemiatry spreads from that small European country which is outstanding not only medically but also politically, economically, culturally, and scientifically: the Netherlands. The great successor of Paracelsus during the seventeenth century, the Flemish nobleman Jean Baptiste van Helmont (1577–1644), equally a chemist, equally a mystic, equally a controversialist, does not abstain from criticism even of his example Paracelsus. In the writings of van Helmont theological and polemic discussions predominate. Van Helmont throws out the whole old humoralism with its bleeding, cauterizing, blisters, fontanelles, clysters, revulsions, and derivations. His goal is to find "arcana," which calm and strengthen the archeus which is located in the region of the stomach. In spite of the fact that van Helmont, like Campanella, regards fever as a curative factor, he is nevertheless an active therapist; he wants to be "rector," not only "minister naturae." His therapeutics (extreme sweating, great quantities of antimony as an emetic) are by no means harmless. He also prescribes numerous disgusting substances of animal origin. Interesting is his slogan: curing by "verbis, herbis, and lapidibus" (words, herbs, and stones), and his promotion of "magnetic" wound treatment. He thus used consciously and unconsciously psychotherapeutics.

The next great iatrochemist is Francis de le Boë, called Sylvius (1614–1675), who made Leyden a famous center of clinical teaching. With him disease depends on "continens, contentum, and anima" (i.e., the contents, the receptacle, and the soul). Like van Helmont, he is primarily interested in the digestive tract. He has a humoral theory, but it is a chemical one and new humors like the pancreatic humor, lymph, and saliva appear in it. His therapy is above all destined to fight overacidity, in a more limited way alkalinization. He too is pious, he too uses a great quantity of antimony, he too bleeds rarely. Because of his frequent use of opiates he received the nickname "Doctor Opiatus."

Ideologically closely related to both these men is M. Ettmüller (1644–1683). His pathology is a typically chemiatric one: bad chylus, lack of ferments, overacidification. Typically chemiatric are also his medicaments: crocus metallicus, tartar emeticus, opiates, iron preparations, mercury. It is interesting that he gives the Peruvian bark in fever and lemon juice in scurvy. His works were well written and therefore widely read. The following notable authors of that period were chemiatrists too: Wedel, Johannes Schroeder, Dolaeus, Schellhammer, Ramazzini, and Vieussens.

Thomas Willis (1621–1675) is the great English chemiatrist. His importance for British and European medicine in the seventeenth century and thereafter has been pointed out recently in a book by H. R. Isler. With Willis, too, the digestive tract is the central problem of pathology. He also frequently uses emetics, one of which bears the fatal name of "Hercules bovis." In discussing drugs Willis mentions the diseases in which they should be used, those in which they should not be used, under any circumstances, and those in which they could be used. This division has been imitated later by many authors. Willis used animal experiment to control drugs. He was the decisive factor in the introduction of the Peruvian bark in England.

Walter Harris (1651–1725), court physician and author of an early book on children's diseases, is a chemiatrist, too. Also regarded as a chemiatrist is Turquet de Mayerne, the Geneva-born French and English court physician. His pharmacopoeia is composed so overwhelmingly of drugs from the plant kingdom that we would rather classify him as an eclectic. Of these soon more.

Riverius, too, although he "introduced chemistry into Montpellier," was rather an eclectic. Abraham Mynsicht (died 1683), the inventor of tartarus emeticus, was an unequivocal prophet of chemiatry.

Besides the men and works just mentioned there exists a great quantity of second-rate chemiatric books like those by Raumelius, Alexander von Suchten, Daelmann, Johannes Hayn, Heinsius, Quercetanus, Bierlinger, Angelisala Vincentinus, etc. Their existence is another proof for the dominating role of chemiatry in the therapeutics of the seventeenth century. Publishers would certainly not have produced such quantities of this literature if there were not a corresponding strong demand. The great influence of chemiatry in the pharmacopoeias of the period, as demonstrated by Urdang, is another piece of evidence for the predominance of chemiatry.

The materials used by historians of pharmacy (inventories, price lists, pharmacopoeias) offer probably the best opportunities to make the above point. In an outstanding monograph, *Die pharmazeutisch-chemischen Produkte deutscher Apotheken im Zeitalter der Chemiatrie* (Bremen, 1957), Gerald Schröder has demonstrated with these materials the advancement of chemiatric products between 1600 and 1670 at the expense of drugs from the vegetable kingdom. In spite of this advance of chemiatry many (e.g., Broen, J. A. Schmitz) did not adopt the new creed. To the extent that the chemiatric drugs were more potent than the Galenic herbs, they were correspondingly more dangerous.

The iatrophysicists, leading especially in Italy, are important as scientists but less influential and less interesting as therapists. In their daily practice they differ very little from the traditionalists. For them too bloodletting is the main weapon. They only interpret it differently, as they are partisans of the Harveyan discovery of the blood circulation. The Harveyan discovery brings about two important new therapeutic inventions by iatrophysicists: blood transfusion (Lower, Denis) and intravenous injection (Wren, Mayor, Elsholz). Both have to be abandoned soon on account of their detrimental side effects, and they return only during the nineteenth centry (see the publications of Heinrich Buess).

As always in history, a large group oscillates between the old and the new, and tries to find a compromise with the different new tendencies: the so-called eclectics. The first author to be mentioned amongst them is Daniel Sennert (1572–1637), who is generally remembered as a fighter against uroscopy. He tries to coordinate the old humoralism and the new chemiatry. Theoretically he puts experience above "ratio," theoretically he praises chemistry (he wrote a textbook of chemistry), practically he uses typical chemiatric drugs like antimony or mercury very often. Nevertheless his pharmacopoeia as a whole consists of the traditional herbs and his subdivision according to four degrees of cold and warm is typically Galenic. He takes over from Sylvius the differentiation between external and internal senses. He is one of the very few who propagate hygienic measures, which he correctly calls an "ars negligata" (a neglected art). In this respect he is continued at the end of the century only by Ramazzini. A Scot living in Poland, John Jonston (1603–1675) follows Sennert in a much-read book which, in an edition by Bonet (1620–1689), existed into the next century. It is typical that in the Bonet edition more metallic drugs are found than in the original Sennert-Jonston book, also far more chemiatric theories, such as the acidity theory of Ettmüller. Peruvian cortex also has entered the book.

Sylvius' disciple, F. Dekker (1648–1720), is another great eclectic, who reports a great number of his own observations. He is quite explicit about the fact that he wants to bring the old and the new together. The innumerable purgatives and clysters he prescribes (they fill three sevenths of his book) are still sometimes directed against the old "humors." Among the sudorifics (two sevenths of his book) we find many chemiatric substances like antimony, crocus metallicus, iron preparations, but also quinine. Also an eclectic was Stefan Blankaart (1650–1702), who equally preached the middle-of-the-road attitude. He was a Cartesian, i.e., oriented toward physics, but he also subscribed to the acidity theory and the antibleeding attitude of the chemiatrists, and the degrees of "cold" and "warm" of the Galenic tradition. Eclectics were furthermore such widely read therapeutic authors as W. Hoefer (1614–1681), G. Horst, and Barbette.

Many paths led to eclecticism in therapeutics. One was a mixture of humoral pathology and a pathology of solids, as represented by Blasius. Blasius warns against too vehement use of purgation, bloodletting, and opiates. Although he edited Willis, he did not mention the Peruvian bark.

The medicine of the preceding century had been characterized by the invasion of exotic drugs. The most powerful and the most important of all exotic drugs, the Peruvian cortex or "China" bark, from which two hundred years later quinine was extracted, came to Europe during the seventeenth century. It is still not known who discovered the drug in Peru and who brought it between 1633 and 1644 to Europe. The latter accomplishment was probably due to the Jesuits, and the bark was in the beginning very often called "Jesuit bark" or "cardinal's powder." For many fanatic Protestants this was a sufficient reason to reject the bark. In spite of its spectacular successes, the medicament was in the beginning the object of bitter fights. Peruvian bark was a phenomenon that did not fit into the categories of traditional Galenism, and which therefore contributed to the decline of Galenism at least as much as the polemics of the chemiatrists. Peruvian bark cured, although it did not have the necessary Galenic "qualities." Eventually the partisans of the most different schools adopted it after initial hesitations (Sydenham, Willis, Dekker, Lister, Cobe, Borelli, Riverius, Baglivi, Waldschmidt, etc.). Some promoters of the bark, like Morton and Torti, were struck by the fact that the bark did not cure all "fevers," but only so-called intermittent fevers. That made it a specific. The first appearance of a drug with a causal, specific effect in a medicine that otherwise was largely symptomatic was of tremendous fundamental importance, the first realization of a new principle.

The recognition of the Peruvian bark makes clearly visible the empiricist element in the therapeutics of the seventeenth century, which sometimes has been overestimated. The fight for the recognition of ipecac followed a course similar to that for the Peruvian bark. Dutch authors like Blankaart and Bontekoe fought for the therapeutic virtues of tea and Dekker and Ettmüller fought for tobacco. Tea was "cleaning the blood." Tobacco served till a hundred years ago primarily as snuff, i.e., as a so-called sternutative (sneezing drug). Sneezing was supposed to clean the brain of bad humors.

Exotic drugs, especially Peruvian bark, reinforced the Paracelsian idea of specifics: Peruvian bark actually was one. Now even Hippocratists like Sydenham and Baglivi dreamed of specifics. The resistance against exotic drugs was partly of an economic nature. They were extremely expensive. Therefore J. Constant de Rebeque at Lausanne substituted cherry bark for Peruvian bark. The former, of course, did not have the same effect.

The Hippocratists of the preceding century (Ballonius, Vallisnieri, Cesalpino, Johannes Lange, etc.) were traditionalists, who differed from the Galenic traditionalists by having more confidence in the healing power of nature and by therefore being less aggressive therapists. Hippocratism continued in the seventeenth century. Its most famous representative is Thomas Sydenham (1624–1689), the so-called English Hippocrates. Some readers might be surprised that we discuss Sydenham only now. But we believe that this attitude corresponds better to reality than the Sydenham myth which, for different reasons, developed during the eighteenth century. Sydenham had by no means the tremendous influence on his contemporaries with which he has been credited later on.

As a therapist Sydenham was, like Baglivi, Willis, and Rivière, a "vampire," i.e., an excessive bleeder. This in spite of the fact that he assumed the iatrogenic nature of some cases of hysteria and of some cases of dropsy in malaria and regarded too much bleeding and purging as the cause of these complications. His skeptical attitude toward materia medica—"it has grown so much, and produced so little"—did not prevent his intensive abuse of mercury. In syphilitics he tried to obtain a salivation of 4000 ml per day. His chase for a chimeric "methodus medendi" is another expression of his old-fashioned dogmatism. His panacea, horseback riding, was the more or less harmless caprice of an old Cromwellian cavalry captain. This panacea was still recommended by Frank and Hufeland. Sydenham's finest therapeutic accomplishment, the adoption of the Peruvian bark, is actually derived from Willis. Sydenham "warmed" his patients with young boys or kittens.

In choosing his drugs, Sydenham was clearly influenced by iatrochemists like Willis, as is evident from his use of crocus metallorum and iron preparations. Sydenham was beyond any doubt, partly on account of his deficient classic education and his previous military-political career, a very able clinician and a relatively able therapist. But the exclusiveness with which he has been studied as the clinician of the seventeenth century has brought about a disfiguration of the medical history of this period. Walter Pagel is, to my knowledge, through his book on van Helmont (1930), the only medical historian of the first half of the twentieth century who escaped the influence of the Sydenham myth.

At this point the problem arises whether, during the seventeenth century, we can still speak of a European medicine or therapeutics, or whether the political-economical formation of national states did not influence medicine to such an extent that such generalizations as European medicine become problematic.

During the seventeenth century another tendency developed, which was to become very important during the following century: therapeutic skepticism. The precursor of this tendency is Daniel Ludwig (1625–1680), who fought with great enthusiasm against too numerous, foul-tasting, expensive, and harmful drugs and for simple drugs. Daniel Ludwig attacks not only single worthless remedies, as Diemerbroeck had done in the case of precious stones. Ludwig goes much farther. In his opinion the number of remedies could easily be reduced to one twelfth or even to one twentieth of those used at present. Although he uses chemiatric medicaments such as antimony and iron, he finds the chemiatrists just as guilty of overmedication as the traditionalists. All this sounds very good. Unfortunately Ludwig's success was limited by the fact that, when his turn came to recommend medicaments, he too recommended such incredible quantities that his own criticism was devaluated. In close relation with skepticism develops, of course, the "expectative method," recommended, e.g., by Gideon Harvey in 1689 in a book carrying the same name.

A reform of therapy was absolutely necessary. The polypharmacy and polypragmasy of the seventeenth century are literally indescrib-

able. Morton, a rather moderate practitioner, gives, e.g., the following treatment of pulmonary tuberculosis on 20 pages of his book
dealing with phthisis. He prescribes repeated bloodletting (6 to 8
ounces in the first stage). Then repeated emetics (3 different prescriptions). Then continuously opiates (4 prescriptions) and regu-
larly purgatives (4 prescriptions). The diaphoretics are indicated (4
prescriptions). A vesicatorium has to be put on the arm or between
the shoulder blades. The stomach needs "lubricantia" and "incrassan-
tia" (9 prescriptions). Balsamic medicaments directed against cough
are necessary (5 prescriptions). Pure, dry air, a light diet, no heavier
beverages than beer, light movements, no excitement or tiresome
thinking are other necessities. This for the first stage. The treatment
of the second and third stages corresponds to the follies of the first.
The famous pharmacopoeias of M. Charas and N. Lemery, or practically any therapeutic publications of the seventeenth century, show
a no less depressing picture (see Alfred Franklin, *Les Médicaments,*
Paris, 1891). One shudders when reading these reports and is
continuously surprised by the toughness of the human constitution.
The polypharmacist Lemery has the merit to have shown that traditional alchemist pyrotechnical methods are insufficient to isolate the
active substances from plants.

The works of Paullini concerning the "Dreckapotheke" (1696)
and medical flagellation (1698) are far more characteristic for the
seventeenth century than the first, modest beginnings of a very hesitant skepticism. Medical flagellation was a strange therapeutic fashion
of the seventeenth century, which was examined in the Zurich Institute in 1963 by Dr. A. Schwarz. In his book on flagellation, i.e.,
therapeutic beating in different diseases, Paullini only compiled
publications of very respected physicians like Meibom and Bartholinus. This form of therapeutics is still found in Trousseau in the
nineteenth century! The mentally sick were in any case beaten, down
to the time of Pinel and Tuke. On that pole of medical thought that
is opposed to skepticism, credulity, the seventeenth century has really
established records, particularly disgusting records. And one should
not blame everything on poor Paullini. Centipedes were after all the
favored medicament of Willis, earthworms that of Ludwig, horse
apples that of Ettmüller. Bartholinus, one of the co-discoverers of the
lymphatic system, prescribed amulets, and others still recommended,

as a consequence of a misinterpretation of a Hippocratic aphorism, castration against rheumatism, gout, leprosy, epilepsy, and mania (see Cabanès, *Remèdes d'autrefois,* Paris, 1910). There were numerous physicians, like R. Fludd, who regarded disease as a consequence of sin and whose main therapy consisted of prayers. There were also astrological physicians like Culpepper. These had studied in universities. Even more lively were the non-academic quacks, whose activity unfortunately we cannot describe here in detail. The kings of France and England meddled in medicine and cured scrofulosis by laying on of hands. This rite was also practiced by ordinary civilians, like the Irish adventurer Greatrake. The noble ex-pirate Digby and many others still prescribed the notorious "sympathetic" wound ointment. Surgery did not advance, but obstetrics continued to progress with van Deventer and Mauriceau.

In 1620 appears the *Novum organum* of Francis Bacon. Therewith begins the long lineage of modern philosophers of experience. But just the example of Bacon shows that the way from a philosophy of experience to well-organized effective experience is a long one. Bacon expresses the wish that his method of induction should also be applied to medicine. He propagates the experiment, which becomes a real fashion during the seventeenth century, but does not look at it uncritically. He calls certain contemporary experiments (probably he is aiming here at alchemists) blind and stupid. He deems vague experiments worthless and unsystematic experience stultifying. His rediscovery of the necessity of repeated experiences and of reporting negative results is remarkable. Yet his own application of his methods did not yield practical results. The same holds true for the prominent Italian iatrophysicist Baglivi. Baglivi was strongly influenced by Bacon, but through his blind admiration of ancient literature fell back behind the consequently anti-Aristotelian Bacon. The famous German clinician Sennert inserts in his *Institutiones* a chapter on the methods of examining the force of medicaments. The contents are rather poor, but he says rightly that experience is more important than theorizing and that it is necessary to observe in men. Such observations should be repeated, only one medicament should be used, and only simple diseases should be observed. I could not find in his writings any traces of his applying his own principles.

Besides the uncontrolled clinical experiment, the animal experiment is often used during the seventeenth century. Only rarely (as in the case of Harvey) is it successful. Intravenous injection is found by animal experiment, but has to be abandoned on account of its failures. The toxicological experiments of Wepfer, who was a very able therapeutic eclectic, are still regarded as exemplary by Pinel more than a hundred years later. The excellent animal experiments with medicaments, which Willis made, are strangely enough forgotten, like so many other of his accomplishments.

During the seventeenth century we observe more therapeutic measures influenced by actual clinical experiments, but dogmatic therapeutics remain still dominant. We see a slow evolution of a theory of experience and of animal experiments. All these tendencies remain yet those of a minority.

IX

Therapeutics in the
Eighteenth Century

THE THERAPEUTICS of the eighteenth century are again dominated by eclecticism, i.e., a chaotic mixture of chemiatric and Galenistic practices which are interpreted partly on the basis of humoral
pathology, partly on the basis of a pathology of solids (fiber or
nervous pathology). Inside and outside of eclecticism we observe a
strengthening of Hippocratic tendencies, i.e., expectative tendencies
confident of the healing power of nature, and of therapeutic skepticism. On the other hand, we note a very dangerous therapeutic
activism, which is mostly presented as a "reform." The publication of
numerous apologies of medicine shows that medicine is passing
through a certain crisis, that confidence in medicine is shaken.
But it is less the medicaments themselves than their application that
is criticized. The mad desire of the eighteenth century to systematize
is not always conducive to reasonable therapeutics.

Enlightenment, the great philosophical trend of the eighteenth
century, influences therapeutics not only in the sense that the pharmacopoeias are relieved of magic and ineffective medicaments,
but also in the sense of adoption of useful folk remedies. An increasing tendency toward empiricism, partly even a true experimentalism,
is observable.

The Leyden professor Herman Boerhaave (1668–1738), the most
famous European physician of the first half of the eighteenth century, was an eclectic. This probably was the basis of his tremendous
reputation. Boerhaave justified his therapeutics by iatrophysical
ideas, like those of the "relaxed fiber," as well as by iatrochemical
theories, like the "lack of acid." As a harmonious personality he
opposed brutal fashions in therapeutics and showed a definite Hippocratic trend toward expectation. Pinel reproached him that he
treated expectatively not only acute but also chronic diseases. Boerhaave recommended the use of harmless plants and fruits. He frequently prescribed opium, one of the few drugs then known that
were objectively effective.

He remained a child of his time with prescriptions that had no
less than forty-four elements, or with such traditional peculiarities as
the prescription of women's milk, bucks' blood, pearls, and so-called
crayfish eyes. Spices served him frequently as medicaments. He prescribed frequently mercury and tartar emetic, often as purgatives.
He was not much opposed to venesections. In this respect he fol-

lowed Sydenham, whom he admired tremendously and whose panacea, horseback riding, he equally adopted. He did not believe in the
existence of specifics. Like his contemporaries Mead, Huxham, and
Heberden, he still favored the so-called fontanelles.

The most famous German physician of the period, Frederic Hoffmann (1660–1742), professor of medicine in Halle, was a well-known
chemist, but explained diseases in the last instance as disturbances
in the hydraulics of the nerve juices. He had not yet abandoned
the idea that nervous diseases could be caused by the devil.
But as a therapist he was extremely sober. He recommended the
reduction of the whole pharmacopoeia to ten or twelve medicaments. It is obvious that the so-called Hoffmann's drops, his invention, was to be one of the twelve survivors. He too made "fontanelles."
His propositions on how to find the effect of a curative plant are
the same as those of Galen. In the case of venesection he did not
take a firm stand. At times he opposed venesection and sweating; at
other times he calls venesection divine. His Hippocratic-skeptical
tendencies are reflected in his strong recommendation of mineral
waters as medicaments. Water became for him a panacea.

His Halle colleague and competitor, G. E. Stahl, the inventor of
the "phlogiston" and the "animism" theories, is well known as the
great promoter of vitalism. He was a firm partisan of expectation, on
which he wrote a book, and prescribed only few, mostly evacuating
drugs. In another book, on chemical medicaments, he is rather
against such. He even opposed the use of Peruvian bark, of iron and
of opium, as he considered these substances too dangerous.

In his *Examinations of Mishandled Diseases* (1726) he dealt in
detail with the abuse of these as well as other medicaments, and
with the spa cures so fashionable during the eighteenth century. Not
only his numerous disciples but also the Hippocratists of Montpellier, who were strongly influenced by him, were inclined toward
expectation. Under his influence the conviction that mental factors
have a disease-producing as well as a curative effect spread more and
more. He still used amulets (against hemoptysis). The successor of
Boerhaave, Gaubius, was equally skeptical. He developed an idea,
found in Hippocrates, and very valuable for future development,
that one has to differentiate between the effect of disease causes and
the reactions of the organism. In order to save the idea of the healing

power of nature, Hoffmann, Stahl, and Gaub regarded many pathological phenomena as "error," as either a too weak or a too strong
reaction of the body. This idea had been uttered before them, e.g.,
by Sydenham and Bohn. Later on we find it in the poet Friedrich
Schiller, who had studied medicine, J. P. Frank, Hecker, Hufeland, F. E. Beneke, and Schoenlein.

While with Sylvius and Boerhaave Leyden had been the center
of Western medicine, now for a number of decades the Edinburgh
medical faculty, developed by Boerhaave pupils, became the center
of European medicine. The best-known therapist of the Scottish school,
William Cullen—his most important work appeared in 1781—was
an eclectic like Boerhaave. He was even more of a Hippocratist. He
was, e.g., more reserved toward venesection. One third of his book
on therapeutics deals with nutrition. Diet was also in the center of
the therapeutic propositions of another noted Anglo-Saxon therapist of this period, G. Cheyne, who in diet recommended invigorat-
ing Peruvian bark, iron, and bathing cures.

The drugs used by Cullen were about the same as those used by
Boerhaave. Opium, wine, and camphor he deemed very important.
He used a little more of the metallic medicaments. Cold water he
regarded as an important help. It is significant for the period, as for
Cullen himself, that he experimented with drugs as well as with
bloodletting. Although Cullen based his pathology on a so-called
neurosis theory of diseases, which he had derived from the experimental physiology and fiber doctrine of Albrecht von Haller, these
theories little influenced his sober therapeutics.

Nothing of this moderation is found in the work of his faithless
pupil, John Brown (1735–1788), who posed as a great reformer.
In his famous *Elementa* (1780) he divided in a very primitive
fashion, the well-known one of the methodists, all diseases into two
kinds, the sthenic ones, produced by too strong stimuli, and the asthenic ones, produced by too weak stimuli. According to him most
diseases were asthenic and had to be treated very actively with
stimulants. His main medicaments, used very generously by himself,
were alcohol and opium. Part of the tremendous success of Brownism, or Brunonianism, which is otherwise hard to understand,
probably has to be attributed to the charms of these drugs. The
armamentarium of Brown contained also the notorious calomel, about

which Brown's American disciple, Benjamin Rush, once made a remark in which there is perhaps more truth than he intended. He called it the "Samson of medicine." Samson did indeed slay great numbers of Philistines.

The teaching of Brown, attractive in its simplicity, found little acclaim in Great Britain, but all the more in Germany, Austria, the United States, and Italy. Girtanner of St. Gallen plagiarized Brown without hesitation in 1790. In Germany, Brownism became particularly popular with Romantics like Roeschlaub (also a great bleeder) and Burdach. But even a Joseph Frank, A. F. Hecker, Weikart, or Reil (Reil turned eventually to Romanticism) adopted it. The Italian version of Brunonianism was promoted by Moscati and Rasori.

It seems that the practical consequences of Brownism were catastrophic, although he did not "evacuate." H. Haeser claims that in the Austrian army, of 600 wounded 400 died within 21 days inebriated, that in the Prussian army after Jena the officers died intoxicated by Rhine wine, the ordinary soldiers intoxicated by ordinary spirits. Rothschuh has shown that the so-called neuropathology and irritation doctrine brought about the complete abandonment of diet.

The Boerhaave pupils van Swieten and de Haen had created a great medical center in Vienna, the so-called Viennese school. They were, like their master and like the most eminent of their successors, Johann Peter Frank, eclectics. Van Swieten is famous for his sublimate treatment of syphilis, which he learned from A. N. Ribeiro Sanchez. Otherwise he was, like his teacher, a traditionalist eclectic, who bled, purged, gave emetics, theriac, etc. Although de Haen criticized the vampirism of Chirac, he was himself a very aggressive bleeder. Probably the most important therapeutic events in the Viennese school were the experiments of Anton Stoerck (1731–1803), which found much attention. He began to publish them at the same time that he became physician of the emperor (1760). Like many of his contemporaries, he was looking for effective medicaments, especially against cancer and mental disease. He tried to find such in going back to substances like hemlock, aconite, the thorn apple (*Datura stramonium*), *Colchicum autumnale*, etc., which either had never become parts of the official pharmacopoeia or had been forgotten.

He began to experiment with hemlock in cancer. He used a methodology which seemed foolproof, in giving the drug first in the animal experiment, then in the self-experiment, and eventually to the patient. Nevertheless his much praised results were worthless. Unfortunately, in spite of his great intelligence, he completely lacked a critical attitude. The number of patients he treated was much too small to draw far-reaching conclusions. Whenever a patient died, he interpreted the sad fact out of existence, in arguing that it was not the disease, but bad weather, consumption of wine, bad general status, which had killed the patient. Some cases, which were errors in diagnosis, were of course cured. Only errors in diagnosis can explain the numerous reports of "cancer cures" by honorable authors, as we find them up to the middle of the nineteenth century.

Stoerck very rapidly developed a tendency to use his drugs as panaceas. Quite naïvely he believed that datura gave him good results in epilepsy and mania. His only real success was the reintroduction of colchicine in the treatment of gout. At the same time another famous Viennese physician, Leopold Auenbrugger, the inventor of percussion, experimented with "psychopharmaca." He used camphor against mania. The Stoerck disciple Collin also gave very high doses of camphor. He "cured" tuberculosis with bloodwort. During the same period belladonna became famous as a cancer drug. It was impossible to maintain this claim, but since this time belladonna has not disappeared from our pharmacopoeias, as other successful uses for it have been found.

During the 1770s emetics, especially tartar emetic, became popular again through the influence of another leader of the Viennese school, the clinician Stoll. Stoerck and Tissot had already recommended emetics. Stoll justified the use of this medication, which he used along with Peruvian bark and artificial vesicants, by the "bilious constitution" of this period. He himself abandoned this method, as he had to realize that it was unsuccessful. He explained this by a change in the "epidemic constitution." Now he turned toward vampirism, i.e., unbridled bloodletting, which he applied to himself. As he suffered from pulmonary tuberculosis, this brought about his early demise. The famous medical historian Haeser reports rather critically on these activities and quotes sources for this period, which claim that in places where there were few physicians, especially few Brownians, mortality was lower, and that later a lower mortality was caused not so much by a change of the "epidemic constitution" as by a less aggressive therapeutic polypragmatism.

The acme of therapeutic mania was reached by the Italian reformer Giovanni Rasori (1766–1837), clinician in Milan, who united in his system bleeding, emetics, and calomel, and called it contrastimulo. Rasori reports himself that he had bled a woman patient, dying at thirty-one, during the last four years of her life 1309 times. And Rasori did this in spite of the fact that he was a very intelligent and decent man. It must also be said that he and his disciples were by no means the only representatives of vampirism and polypharmacy in this period. As eminent an eclectic as Goethe's friend Hufeland based his therapeutics on the three "heroes," i.e., venesection, emetics, and opium. With these heroes he treated, e.g., the widespread pulmonary tuberculosis. While many leaders of medicine continued energetically to preach venesection, the voices against bleeding and its abuse became more and more frequent (e.g., Wolstein, F. X. Mezler). Clysters were and remained less controversial, although they were no longer quite as popular as during the seventeenth century. Our criticism of hyperactive therapeutic methods would be ahistorical if there had not been simultaneously, as well as before and afterward, representatives of less dangerous forms of therapeutics.

The eighteenth century has been properly called the century of Enlightenment, and the philosophy of Enlightenment has influenced medicine in many ways. There are, for example, a number of specialties with their early forms of therapeutics, such as psychiatry, orthopedics, pediatrics, industrial medicine, and veterinary medicine, which came into being in connection with the philosophy of Enlightenment. In the field of therapeutics two phenomena are above all typical for Enlightenment medicine: the cleaning of pharmacopoeias through elimination of magic and inefficient remedies, and the unprejudiced examination and adoption of folk remedies. Between 1748 and 1758 the Paris "Code" was purged of substances that seemed to be of magic origin. In 1748 the last edition of Paullini's *Dreckapotheke* appeared. In 1745 Heberden had published his famous pamphlet against mithridaticum and theriac. Haller praises, in his preface to the Basle pharmacopoeia (1771), the reduction of the hypertrophic Britannic pharmacopoeia, which followed Heberden's courageous step. R. A. Vogel gives long lists of obsolete medicaments in his *Historia materiae medicae* (1760). The zeal of the reformers sometimes went too far, when, e.g., they eliminated useful drugs like opium, quinine, iron, mercury, belladonna, and hyoscyamus, because these drugs had once been used in a magic connection. Typical for the change is *An Explanation of the New Austrian Military Pharmacopoeia,* which appeared in 1800. This book describes 92 drugs that had been discussed in the old pharmacopoeia, 47 that had been added, and 154 that had been eliminated. In 1808, J. J. Loos wrote a whole book on such eliminated drugs. The noted clinician Tronchin from Geneva, a favorite disciple of Boerhaave, owed his great reputation largely to the fact that he condemned the greater part of all drugs. The same attitude made the phrenologist Gall a most popular physician in Vienna as well as in Paris. It is probably no accident that in this period the word "placebo" was introduced into medical language; i.e., insight into the real nature of drug use had increased considerably. To a certain extent these phenomena are a continuation of the older skepticism of Hoffmann and others, or reflections of the Rousseau doctrine, "Back to nature."

It is therefore not surprising that simultaneously with the abandonment of useless and disreputable drugs, treatment by bathing was revived. We mentioned Hoffmann for earlier attempts in this direction. A great promotor of bathing and spas was the renowned Bordeu of Montpellier, who was also a friend of theriac. Aix in Savoy was rediscovered as a spa. Spa in Belgium became the fashionable center. Hydrotherapeutics was recommended by Floyer, the Hahns, Currie, Pomme, and others. Heliotherapeutics flourished especially in France in the 1770s with Faure, Lapeyre, Bertrand, and others. In England the first colonies for scrofulous children at the sea coast were opened, where they were to receive sun and sea baths. Gymnastics was again honored through the work of Fuller, C. J. Tissot, Bordeu, Helvetius, Gutsmuths, Clias, and others. Diet again found greater attention (Unzer, S. A. Tissot, Zückert, et al.). The thinkers of the Enlightenment also proved the nonsensical nature of the notion of panacea. But the word of Balzac's friend, Dr. Naquart, of 1819 is probably still valid: "The faith in panaceas, it seems, is today rather disguised than that it has died out."

The other specific tendency of the Enlightenment is the adoption of folk remedies after evaluation of their actual efficacy. Basically this had been Stoerck's method. This tendency might be connected with the fact that during the Enlightenment, for the first time in medical history, physicians abandoned the aristocratic traditions of medicine and felt responsible to all strata of the population, especially the poor. To treat the poor they needed drugs that were effective as well as cheap. All physicians mentioned in the following were outspoken adherents of Enlightenment. This holds true for Fowler, who introduced the celebrated arsenic preparation into the treatment of fevers (arsenic passed through a period of discredit during the eighteenth century). It is also applicable to Percival, who, in 1771, used cod liver oil, a Scandinavian folk remedy, against rheumatism. In the beginning of the nineteenth century cod liver oil became a remedy against rickets and scrofulosis. Adherents of Enlightenment were also those who introduced ergot and cortex salicis (1762) into official therapeutics. Belladonna had been used since 1720 by surgeons in "cancer cures" and was undoubtedly successful in chronic mastitis. Belladonna was also used against rabies; and Grundig introduced it into the treatment of abdominal pain, Himly into the treatment of eye diseases. In adopting such folk remedies, mistakes were unavoidable, as when Gaub took over from the cobbler Ludemann the zinc treatment of epilepsy.

Digitalis is undoubtedly the most important folk remedy introduced by a partisan of Enlightenment into the pharmacopoeia. Digitalis, growing only in the North, was unknown to the ancients, as was belladonna. Digitalis is mentioned in the works of Fuchs (1543) and Bock (1539) as a folk remedy. It remained one till William Withering identified it in 1775 as the active substance among the twenty-two herbs that were used in a tea of an old woman. In 1785 he published his book on digitalis. Digitalis has remained for a long time one of the very few objectively effective drugs in our pharmacopoeia.

Withering was a remarkable man. Born into a family of doctors in 1741 in Shropshire, he studied in Edinburgh under Cullen and others, became a Freemason, and was an acquaintance of Fowler, whom we have already mentioned. He settled as a country doctor in Stafford and began around 1766 to collect flowers. In 1775 he moved to the very active young industrial town of Birmingham, where he belonged to the Lunar Society, an association of partisans of Enlightenment. In 1776 he published his book *British Plants*, in 1785 his book on digitalis. In 1786 he retired to the country because of pulmonary tuberculosis, which killed him in 1799. In 1790 his city house was, like that of Priestley, sacked by a mob on account of his sympathy for the French Revolution. Withering was active in many branches of social reform (abolition of slavery, fight against alcoholism, against duels), and had an international reputation.

His book on digitalis he published after trying the remedy for ten years. He wanted to avoid its misuse. He reported all his cases, also those with fatal outcomes. First he describes the botanic characteristics and the history of the plant. Color, smell, taste, and chemistry of the plant did in no way explain its specific effectiveness. The same holds for experiments with turkeys or for analogies. The drug had been given against epilepsy, scrofulosis, wounds, and dyspnea. Withering does not believe in any of these indications. For him it is a superb diuretic, a remedy against "dropsy." We should not forget that the different sources of edema were then still unknown. "Dropsy" therefore was not a symptom, but a disease.

Withering reports that he tried the drug first among his poor patients. In the beginning he gave too high doses in the erroneous assumption that, in order to obtain the diuretic effect a certain sickness was necessary. Now he warns against these doses. First he gave decocts, then infusions, and eventually the powder. The drug was successful with him in ascites, anasarca, dropsy of the chest. He did not believe in its value in pulmonary tuberculosis (phthisis). He reports in detail 170 cases, mostly so-called asthma (probably identical with our cardiac asthma). It is striking how many bad cases of alcoholism are among his patients. Besides his own cases he quotes letters of 14 other physicians who had tried the drug. One of them, Jones, had statistically analyzed his 24 cases.

Withering realized that the drug did not work in all dropsies, but only in certain "constitutions." He called it a diureticum, but he was aware of the fact that the medicament very strongly influenced the heart and that it had no effect in so-called hard edema, in isolated ascites, or in dropsy of the ovary, which, since the time of Galen, were all classified as dropsies. Withering mentioned in his book everything that could be said about the medicament, considering that dropsy had not yet been separated into its different elements and shown to be only a symptom. He cannot be reproached for not having known or recognized these connections. A later description of the further history of digitalis, which was immediately used by many as a panacea, will show how valuable were the results Withering obtained in this field without refined methods, through simple, thorough, and honest observation.

We have dealt in the preceding in somewhat more detail with Withering on account of the value of his personality as well as because of the value of the drug he discovered.

Another folk remedy was citrus fruits, introduced by Lind in the treatment and prevention of scurvy on the basis of a famous controlled experiment. Lind's experiments of May 20, 1747, mark in a double sense an epoch in the history of therapeutics. First, it was of the greatest importance to obtain eventually a clearly effective weapon against scurvy, which was particularly widespread and murderous amongst sailors. The English owe to his discovery partially their victory over Napoleon. Second, from the point of view of bringing about greater objectivity in therapeutic experience, the introduction of the controlled experiment by Lind was a historic turning point.

During the so-called Continental Blockade of Napoleon, a great many native remedies were examined in Europe for obvious reasons. Neither this movement nor similar ones during the American Civil War or in Hitler's Third Reich yielded positive results.

Lind's loan from folk medicine belongs not only to the field of curative medicine but also to the field of prevention. The most important folk preventive adopted by official medicine was the inoculation with cowpox introduced by Jenner. Jenner, a country physician, had heard about this technique from farmers and their female servants. Jenner's discovery came at the end of a century that had learned earlier to prevent pox by the so-called inoculation learned from the Turkish heathens.

Inoculation and vaccination played an enormous role in Enlightenment medicine. Their defense and their application are typical, almost "pathognomonic" for the true Enlightenment physician, whether he be court physician, professor, or simple practitioner. They are as typical for the men of Enlightenment as antimony was once for the chemiatrists.

Both methods of immunization, variolation and vaccination, are only the most visible part of the mentality of prevention that penetrates the whole medicine of Enlightenment, and has found its classical expression in the works of Tissot and Johann Peter Frank. Prevention is more effective than, as well as, in the long run, cheaper than. treatment. Characteristic of the therapeutics of Enlightenment are the evolution of orthopedics (which is closely connected with the foundation of a home for crippled children in Orbe, Switzerland, by Venel in 1780), the evolution of scientific pediatrics (the book by Rosen von Rosenstein was published in 1764), and the evolution of scientific psychiatry.

We mentioned previously that with Stahl psychogenesis and psychotherapy officially entered into science during the 18th century. Publications concerning psychogenesis were those by Ludwig, Zückert, Harper, Fischer, and Langermann; publications concerning psychotherapy were those by Bolten, Scheidemantel, Tissot, Falconer, Haslam, Reil, and Bordeu. The greatest psychotherapist of the century was Philippe Pinel. The so-called animal magnetism, introduced by Mesmer in 1774, was intended to be a physical, magnetic treatment, but actually it was psychotherapeutics. Psychotherapeutics was actually also exorcism, which some Romantic physicians, like Justinus Kerner, tried to reintroduce at the end of the century.

Enlightenment brought a changed attitude toward secret remedies. Secret remedies have always existed, whether they were those of the medicine man, the stamp-guaranteed Roman secret remedies, ridiculed by Lukian, or those of the alchemists. A detailed description of the secret remedies of the seventeenth century can be found in Hermann Schelenz's *History of Pharmacy,* page 522 et seq. For those of the eighteenth century see in the same volume page 578 et seq., and for those of the nineteenth century see page 642 et seq. and 768 et seq.; also see Franklin (1891, pages 207–237) and Cabanès (1910, page 433 et seq.). Grete de Francesco has left us a very fine book on the charlatans of the seventeenth and eighteenth centuries. The more recent history of secret remedies in the United

States during the last decades has been very thoroughly studied by James Harvey Young in his *Toadstool Millionaires* and *Medical Messiahs.*

Only through Enlightenment did it become generally recognized during the second half of the eighteenth century that secret remedies are unethical. In the beginning of the century the famous Halle clinicians Stahl and Hoffmann sold secret remedies without hesitation. In 1770 John Gregory condemned them energetically. Johann Christian Wilhelm Juncker of Halle published in 1788 the contents of a secret remedy invented by his grandfather, in order to practice what he preached, i.e., the refusal of secret remedies.

There is a close connection between secret remedies and quackery. Quackery is very old, as we have already discussed when reporting the passages of Rhazes. It is possible to speak of quackery in a clearly defined sense only if a canon of medicine more or less guaranteed by government exists. Ever since such "official" physicians have existed, they have bitterly complained about the competition of quacks. Particularly frequent are complaints concerning theologians (e.g., Berkeley, Wesley) and paramedical professions, like apothecaries. There do exist plenty of quacks with an M.D. diploma, as, e.g., the history of the rejuvenation swindles of the last centuries have demonstrated abundantly. The favored domains of the quacks are, of course, diseases that the patient does not like to show to the physician, like venereal diseases, or incurable diseases, like cancer, where the unfortunate victims out of fear are willing to feed the worst crooks. A strange aspect of quackery is that not only does it impress the uneducated lower strata of society, but at the top of the pyramid, among kings and other leaders of this world, quackery has always found numerous friends.

During the eighteenth century Krüger (1744), Kratzenstein (1745), Nollet (1746), and Jallabert from Geneva (1748) made electrotherapy fashionable. Such famous physicians as Linné, Sauvages, De Haen, Marat (who treated society with the guillotine), or laymen like Franklin were interested in electrotherapy. The discoveries of Galvani (1791) and Alexander von Humboldt reinforced this therapeutic trend, on which Curt Sprengel has reported extensively. Another fashionable treatment became, after 1770, that with the newly discovered oxygen, which was recommended above all by Fourcroy and Beddoes. These two new discoveries promptly degenerated into panaceas. In connection with the progress of chemistry, innumerable unsuccessful attempts were made to find a solvent for bladder stone.

One of the great therapeutic heresies in medical history, homeopathy, is a child of the late eighteenth century. The criticism of its founder, Hahnemann, concerning the therapy of his days, especially unlimited bleeding, was perfectly legitimate and found a tremendous echo. His own recommendations were meant to be no less activistic. But in view of the enormous dilution of his medicaments his treatment actually meant that the physician lets nature take its course. When the first therapeutic statistics were drawn up, the patients of the homeopaths did better than the anemic and antimony- and mercury-poisoned patients of the allopaths. It took some time till the allopaths were as therapists objectively superior to the homeopaths.

Deserving mention in this context is that the scientific, practical, and social rise of surgery in France as well as in Great Britain during the eighteenth century was quite extraordinary. We would like to remind our reader here only of the names of Jean Louis Petit, Desault, Charles White, and John Hunter.

The influence of religious motivations in therapeutics is clearly illustrated by the different scientific opinions of British (Protestant) and French (Catholic) obstetricians concerning Caesarian section as laid down during this century. The French, who, as Catholics, had to baptize the child above all, were far more inclined to operate than the economy-minded Protestant Englishmen, who were primarily interested in the conservation of the more expensive mother. F. Brupbacher has shown in the twentieth century that in a similar fashion the medical indication of abortion in tuberculosis was a function of birth statistics: the greater the number of births, the more abortion was indicated in this disease.

The eighteenth century produced a theoretician of medical experience, Johann Georg Zimmermann of Brugg, Switzerland, whose book on this subject was published in 1763. In classic form he unmasks what he calls "false experience": "In general, experience is regarded to be the knowledge of a thing which one has looked at frequently. According to these criteria a man who has traveled a great deal has the greatest experience of the world. An old officer has the greatest experience of the art of warfare. An old nurse of medicine. . . . One sees that this false experience is nothing else but the lawless, old, or blind routine. . . . The crowd confuses the practice of the medical art with the ordinary practice of a craft; it confuses a science of the spirit with a dexterity of the fingers."

Pinel, though very strongly influenced by Zimmermann, said somewhat ironically: "In general it is much easier to indicate the traps one should avoid than to indicate with precision the road one should follow." This holds true for Zimmermann. He looks through pseudoexperience, which in reality is but routine. The critical attitude of the Enlightenment thinkers against the guild-ridden craftsmen (we find similar remarks in Diderot's encyclopedia or with J. Chr. W. Juncker) enables him to some extent to see that much of this craftsmen "experience" (also in agriculture) is fossilized pseudoexperience. Some of so-called experience even is unmasked as pure superstition. But Zimmermann is too much of a bookworm to find more than a verbal answer for his problem: "Experience needs genius." It is amazing that Zimmermann, who, together with Haller, had made numerous animal experiments, rarely mentions these in this connection. Haller himself discussed in his pharmacopoeia introduction, not animal experiments, but clinical experiments in hospitals. Until those are made, Haller recommends *"paucissima fides"* (very little confidence).

In Germany numerous discussions of the "Methodology of the Examination of Drugs" were published. The real practical progress in the field of objective examination of therapeutic experience during the eighteenth century was realized in England. It is probably no accident that this country, changed through the revolutions of the seventeenth century, remains during the eighteenth century the land of the philosophy of experience (Locke, Hume, the Millses) and progresses also greatly in the field of economics and politics. The philosopher Berkeley had suggested controlled clinical experiments. The real founder of this extremely important method is James Lind. In his famous scurvy experiments of May 20, 1747, he submitted twelve scurvy patients to six different methods of treatment and could prove easily the superiority of citrus fruits. Adoption of the controlled clinical experiment, a thing of decisive importance, was very slow. As late as 1851 Wunderlich condemned it as unethical, and Fonssagrives in the *Dictionary of Dechambre* does not mention it in 1874 when enumerating the methods of examining drugs. The introduction of inoculation and vaccination against smallpox created, during the eighteenth century, numerous opportunities for controlled clinical experiments (e.g., by Sloane, Jenner, J. P. Frank). In 1760, Daniel Bernoulli proved, by the theory of probabilities, the value of inoculation.

In the field of therapeutic animal experiments, deserving particular mention are those of Browne Langrish (1746) with cherry laurel water. Langrish showed real insight into the fact that animal experiments have to be undertaken in sufficient numbers and that negative results have to be reported. The same holds for the opium experiments of Fontana, which, beyond any doubt, are the best in the long series of opium experiments of the eighteenth century undertaken by Haller, Whytt, Monod, Alston, and others. The frequency of opium experiments is probably connected with the frequency of the use of opium during this period. The majority of animal experiments with drugs during the eighteenth century, as reported by P. Bernkopf in 1936, unfortunately do not show any of these methodological insights. Most of these toxicological examinations were made only once with the same substance in one animal.

It is most regrettable that pharmacological experiments with human blood in vitro, undertaken during the eighteenth century and reported by Lindenberger in 1937, had a point of departure that condemned them to failure. The results of such in vitro experiments are irrelevant for practical therapeutics. Otherwise some of the authors analyzed by Lindenberger, like John Freind (1675–1728) or J. T. Eller (1689–1760), are, as far as the thoroughness of their experiments and their number are concerned, progressive and exemplary.

During the late eighteenth century the pharmacological-therapeutic works of the great Viennese clinician A. Stoerck, discussed previously, were tremendously admired. Today they rather serve as an example that a researcher cannot obtain good results, even with good and progressive methods, if his critical judgment is submerged by enthusiasm. Withering, on the other hand, showed that, even with very simple methods, valid results can be obtained. The greater the objectivity with which experiences are reported, the more discussions around "principles" and "systems" are transformed into discussions around technical details. This evolution becomes quite visible in the eighteenth century.

X

Therapeutics at the Beginning of the Nineteenth Century: Traditionalism, Skepticism, Physiologism

IT IS surprising to see that around the turn of the century and in the first half of the nineteenth century humoralistic-Galenic tradition in therapeutics was, in spite of various and contradictory theories, still very strong. Cabanis was certainly right when stating that nobody claimed any more publicly to be a partisan of Galen, but practically he was still followed very frequently. His humoralism reappears above all disguised as chaotic eclecticism.

Simultaneously therapeutic skepticism became very influential, especially in Paris and Vienna. Under the influence of the skeptics, clinically controlled experiments gained decisive importance. It is strange to see that these therapeutic skeptics, especially in Paris, believed themselves to be but "Hippocratists." Skepticism in Paris was paralyzed for one and a half decades by the murderous reform-activism of J. F. Broussais.

In Paris we observe furthermore that the work of Magendie brings about the beginning of "physiologism," which was destined to become the road toward a new therapeutics. With Magendie the therapeutic animal experiment, experimental pharmacology, became victorious. The numerous new drugs, which chemistry and the study of folk remedies gave to medicine during this period, were immediately and extensively abused.

Humoralism in therapeutics meant above all the permanent use of the unholy trinity: bleeding, emetics, and cathartics. Blood, lung, and gastrointestinal tract, etc., were still "cleaned." Things had even grown worse, as the Galenists had mixed, since the seventeenth century, with the chemiatrists and now used as emetics such toxic substances as antimony, and as cathartics the equally toxic calomel. It should not be forgotten that even in the "skeptic" Paris of 1828 an epidemic of acrodynia—i.e., iatrogenic mercury poisoning—broke out. Typical for the prevalence of humoralistic ideas is that it was still regarded as dangerous to treat certain skin diseases, hemorrhoids, fever, gout, etc., because the corrupted humors would then attack the internal organs (see, for example, the book of D. Raymond, Paris, 1816). The main representatives of these traditionalist therapeutics are the so-called eclectics, like Johann Peter Frank, Hufeland, A. G. Richter, Authenrieth, Romberg, Schoenlein, and Krukenberg in Germany. These eclectics have often been called "rational empiricists." This expression is self-contradictory and reflects a contradictory practice. What patchwork could be produced by such eclectics is shown by A. F. Hecker, who in 1791 still recommended Alexander of Tralles, Fernel, Mercatus, and Sanctorius as guideposts for the practitioner, but at the same time almost completely adopted Brownism. It was possible to state openly, as Reil did, that the old therapeutics (bleeding, emetics, cathartics, baths plus opium and bark) lacked any scientific basis, and yet continue it for "empirical" reasons.

If was, of course, possible to combine eclecticism with sound common sense, like Johann Peter Frank, for example, who very often put his confidence in the healing power of nature or prevention, recommended expectation or psychotherapy, and spoke up against the "poisoning century." Nevertheless, even he was very generous in prescribing bloodletting, emetics, cathartics, fontanelles, etc., and cannot be regarded as a safe practitioner. The situation was worse with those who did not have too much sound common sense at their disposal, like Hufeland, who did not shy away from the application of his three "heroes"—bleeding, emetics and opium—even in the case of pulmonary tuberculosis. And Hufeland firmly believed that he was but a "servant of nature" and an empiricist! And we do not want to deny that his fight against Brunonianism or for hygienic progress, especially cowpox vaccination, was meritorious. The whole brainlessness of this traditionalism became obvious in the cholera epidemics of the century, when the totally dehydrated victims were "treated" with venesection (most of the time no blood came anymore) or calomel.

In 1800 Hufeland wrote the strange sentence, "Each curative measure is an artificial disease," which did not go unnoticed. He made this statement probably under the influence of Hahnemann. For Hahnemann the point of departure of all therapeutic endeavors was the idea of chasing one disease with another. The idea of driving out diseases with diseases is very old. Such "curative" diseases are above all fever, hemorrhages, and eczemas. This idea is found in the Hippocratic writings; it was developed particularly by Rufos and was defended by Galen, out of whose writings it sedimented into folklore. It reappears again more strongly in the seventeenth century in the writings of Solenander and Primrose. Boerhaave was a partisan of this idea, and therefore a whole literature on the "*Morbi*

salutares" (useful diseases) arose in this century. It flourished
particularly in Germany through the writings of Alberti, Baldinger,
Hornung, Richter, Schrader, Weger, Karthäuser, and numerous doctoral dissertations. At the end of the century Mezler, Vigarout, and
Broussonnet even practiced a kind of malaria therapy. In Germany
the idea had a comeback in the twenties of the nineteenth century,
probably in connection with Hahnemann and Hufeland, and then
disappeared for a longer period. In France, too, it had a certain
echo in the second decade of the nineteenth century. Among prominent physicians it was acclaimed primarily by the dermatologist
Rayer.

In this connection we would like to remind the reader of the
fatal theory concerning the value of postoperative suppuration, the
so-called laudable pus. This theory implies that suppuration is necessary for the healing of a wound. This idea existed from Galen to
Lister. Related to the idea that one disease drives out another one is
the theory of the so-called antagonism of certain diseases, which also
was maintained up to the middle of the nineteenth century. It was,
for instance, believed that leprosy and plague, leprosy and syphilis,
leprosy and hemorrhoids, plague and scurvy, phthisis and typhoid
fever, etc., were mutually exclusive.

No less repulsive than the unholy triad of venesection, emetics,
and cathartics was the abuse of drugs, practiced simultaneously,
especially under the influence of Brunonianism. Typical are some
figures taken from the records of the Bamberg hospital, which was
directed by Marcus, one of the leading German Romantic physicians
and Brunonians. In 1798 there were 480 patients in this hospital.
During this year each patient consumed an average of 1 dram of
opium, 195g camphor, 1 ounce of liquor anodynus, 132g serpentaria,
528g Peruvian bark, more than 1 quart of distilled alcohol. In addition
each patient consumed considerable quantities of moschus, naphtha
vitrioli, arnica, valeriana, angelica, cinnamon, tinctura martisonica,
and elixir roburans vitii. This Romantic polypharmacy was combined with metaphysical empty talk, as an ordinary sentence from
J. F. Sobernheim's handbook of practical pharmacology (Berlin,
1838, page 236) might illustrate: "Like all saturnine drugs, sugar
of lead contracts the fiberlike formations, limits and restrains more
or less all animal excretions and secretions, especially the peripheral

functions, and above all arrests the action of the bowels, retards and restrains the pathological activity of serous, phlegm, and pus excreting areas and the action of the lymphatic gland system. By exerting this contracting effect on the vessels and especially on the arterial sphere of them, it tunes down simultaneously the erethism of vessels combined with a pathological, too expansive, orgiastic activity of blood and decomposition and melting of animal material." Typical for the almost unbelievable polypharmacy of this period is that a representative physician like Hufeland in his *Pharmacopoeia for the Poor* (!) of 1812 mentions no less than 550 drugs. Johann Peter Frank was at least satisfied with a minimum of 50 and Sundelin with 100. Even in his *Encheiridion* of 1836, Hufeland still gives 273 prescriptions.

In this period the opposition between "the art" of medicine and medical science was strongly underlined. Up to the eighteenth century art was understood as a craft, therefore also medical art. This craft-art absorbed scientific elements without too great difficulties. The older vitalists thought of themselves as scientists. But when science became predominantly experimental, and science and experimental science menaced to take over medicine, the so-called artists arose against science. J. Chr. W. Juncker, in 1788, carried on a controversy against the "impervious emotions of these poets" in medicine. This "artistic" attitude was, of course, particularly outspoken with the German Romantic physicians, like Ringseis, who raved of the "curing instinct," intuition, and "esthetic sensations" in medicine. The French clinicians, no mystics, but no less enemies of science, preached so-called tact, which they compared to the "taste" of poets and painters, or the "*coup d'oeil,*" which was supposedly a quality of politicians. In the course of the nineteenth century these antiprogressive, divining-rod clinicians were less heard of. But a mighty wave of "curative instinct" arose in Germany after 1918, where in all fields an attempt was made to compensate for the defeat by mystics and metaphysics. Such a relapse into the attitudes of the medicine man is very often financially quite rewarding. "Instinct" cannot be learned, and has therefore to be paid better than knowledge, which can be acquired.

In view of the above-mentioned deplorable situation it was very important—it was actually a decisive turning point in the history of therapeutics—that skepticism, which had so far grown only slowly, was now taken up by prominent clinicians in leading medical centers like Vienna and Paris. In Paris medicine had been transformed, institutionally and as far as content is concerned, in the wake of the Revolution of 1789. Medicine and surgery were reunited. Generalizing humoralism was replaced by localistic solidism, a medicine of symptoms by a medicine of lesions. A new active form of observation, composed of physical examination, autopsy, and statistic analysis, became the basis of a medicine, which I have called hospital medicine, as its evolution can only be understood in connection with the evolution of the hospitals in this period. Hospital medicine was basically different from the preceding bedside, as well as from the following laboratory medicine. This hospital medicine was accompanied in Paris by hospital pharmacy. The many different and interesting aspects of the latter have been described in detail by Alex Berman. The misfortune of this new clinic was that, reacting against the abuses of the past, it refused to use the microscope, chemistry, and experimental physiology. This led later into a dead end. Its most important contribution to therapeutics was therapeutic skepticism, to which all its leaders, with the exception of Broussais and his immediate disciples, subscribed.

In France a certain skeptic, expectative, Hippocratic tradition in medicine did exist before the Revolution with such men as Tronchin, Desbois de Rochefort, Gilibert, Vitet, and Voullonne. Skepticism was also supported by the fashionable slogan of Rousseau: "Back to nature!"

Therapeutic skepticism is not nihilism—i.e., abolition of drug therapy. Radical nihilistic slogans—like that of Piedagnel, "The best treatment is the absence of treatment," or of Andral, "All methods of treatment fail, all methods of treatment succeed"—are very rare in Paris. They can be more often found with Americans who studied in Paris, like E. Bartlett or Oliver Wendell Holmes, or with certain Viennese clinicians. Bartlett recommended the abolition of nine tenths of all drugs. Oliver Wendell Holmes wrote: "I am firmly convinced, that if the whole materia medica, as used now, would be sent to the bottom of the sea, this would be very good for mankind—and very bad for the fishes."

Therapeutic skepticism is not primarily polemizing against the one or the other medicament; it is thorough, nondogmatic examination of all traditional drugs and curative methods, as the therapeutic skepticist suspects many of them to be either ineffective or even detrimental. The therapeutic skeptic is an empiricist. Therapeutic skepticism advocates the reduced employment or even the abolition of drugs and methods that cannot be proven useful. Therapeutic skepticism brings about greater confidence into the healing power of nature. The famous Cuvier wrote rightly that the elimination of bad medicaments is a positive action.

In the history of therapeutics "empirical" and "rational" activities have always been differentiated. While one group of therapists proceeded "rationally"—i.e., based their therapeutics on scientific systems and theories—the other group aimed at processes founded chiefly on direct experience. We have seen in the fourth chapter that this differentiation is very artificial, that so-called rationalists occasionally took experience as their point of departure, and that many empiricists actually proceeded from rational dogmas and were quite deluded concerning the objective character of their "empiricism." It is nevertheless undeniable that Parisian skepticisn put the emphasis on experience and that experience eventually acquired a solid basis in the form of statistics and experiments. The Parisians believed in general that real causal knowledge of diseases is impossible and unnecessary for therapeutics. Therapeutics should, as Cabanis said, not be derived from physiology and pathology, but empirically from therapeutics itself.

The skepticism of the Parisian school was directed primarily against drug therapy. French definitions of therapeutics during this period show that drug therapy was no longer the only form of therapy. It was a return to the definitions of Erasistratus or Galen. Schwilgué, the therapist among the disciples of Pinel, defined therapeutics in 1805 as being either hygiene or materia medica. Gaspard L. Bayle, the therapist amongst the disciples of Corvisart, defined therapeutics as composed of materia medica, surgery, and hygiene. Barbier d'Amiens, who continued the therapeutic work of Bichat, defined therapeutics in 1822 as a combination of hygiene, materia medica, and physical methods. Guersent, the friend of Bretonneau, subdivided therapeutics in 1844 into physics, chemistry, surgery, hygiene (consisting of diet and moral treatment), and eventually materia medica. It is also typical that in the book of Trousseau on therapeutics, diet and gymnastics are the neighbors of metallic prescriptions, opium and digitalis or treatment by heat and cold.

Hygiene was at that time in Paris an ambiguous expression. It could be an equivalent for public health and could also mean individual prevention. It could furthermore be an equivalent for non-medicamentous methods of treatment, like diet, fresh air, warm and cold water, electrotherapy, magnetism, and psychotherapy. It was the most positive aspect of the skeptic reduction of drug treatment that physical methods like gymnastics and baths, surgery including specialized surgery, psychotherapy, preventive medicine, and nursing developed tremendously. It should never be forgotten how greatly good nursing influences the success of therapeutics.

A frequent reproach against the Parisian school is that it was more interested in pathological anatomy than in therapeutics. That it was very much interested in surgery is conveniently forgotten in this context. Rostan answered rightly that "the medicine of symptoms without knowledge of local diagnosis is absurd, powerless, and sometimes detrimental and fatal." This connection between improved diagnostics and improved therapeutics cannot be sufficiently emphasized. Certain verbal acrobats of reform in the beginning of the twentieth century never understood this. Rostan was able to show that during the reign of the new, supposedly not therapeutically oriented medicine the mortality in the Hôtel Dieu, the largest Paris hospital, was from 1789 to 1844 reduced to 50 percent of what it was before the Revolution. The reproach that the Parisian school did not sufficiently practice general treatment and individualization of treatment is more justified. This is connected with the localism of the Parisian school and with its "ontology" (interest centering around disease, not the diseased).

Parisian skepticism was not a panacea, but it was a very necessary and important step toward progress in modern therapeutics. Skepticism leads toward empiricism. One can state that the skeptics of the nineteenth century were the first true empiricists in medical history.

Philippe Pinel, a Hippocratist, educated in Montpellier, from 1795 to 1816 the head of the Parisian school, speaks of a "feeling of utter disgust with polypharmacy." In later editions of his *Philosophical Nosography,* he literally quotes the devastating judgment of his pupil

Bichat, who called the materia medica of the period "an amorphous mixture of imprecise ideas, often childish observations, and delusive resources." His suggestions for a reform were: "Simplify the materia medica to the extreme, limit it to the use of a small number of native plants of known effect, or to simple chemical substances." Pinel searched for a better method to obtain therapeutic experience. He deemed it necessary to treat clearly defined diseases in a controlled environment. Pinel practiced what he preached. In the fight between active and expectative medicine he opted energetically in favor of the latter, having full confidence in the healing power of nature. He hardly ever used venesection or cathartics. He even turned down "poisonous" quinine in the treatment of malaria. He was, on the other hand, a protagonist of smallpox inoculation as well as smallpox vaccination, and other hygienic measures, including psychotherapy. He went much farther than his mentor Cabanis, who preached against vampirism but bled himself extensively and prescribed antimony. Cabanis inaugurated the more modern prescription of iron. Pinel was by no means the only skeptic amongst the early leaders of the Parisian school. Chaussier and Guersent prescribed little, Double cursed the British drug mania, Fouquier was expectative, and Portal always waited five years before using a new remedy.

Bichat, the disciple of Pinel, who, on account of his early death (1802), did not become his heir, has left us in print only a few pages concerning therapeutics. They are contained in the "General Considerations" of his *General Anatomy*. We have already quoted the critical sentence that Pinel took over. The following statement of Bichat's is interesting: "The same medicaments have been used successively by humoralists and solidists. Theories changed, but the medicaments remained the same. They were always used and they had always the same effect. This proves that their effect is independent of the opinions of physicians and that they can be evaluated only through observations." Fortunately the collection of student notebooks of the Zurich Medical Historical Institute contains the notebooks of a Parisian student of 1802, Louis Nicolas Jusserandot, who assisted the last lecture course of Bichat, which could not be finished because of the sudden death of the teacher. This course was devoted to "materia medica." For Bichat his previous anatomical, physiological, and pathological activities had been only preparations for a new therapeutics. Through these notes we are a little better oriented concerning the therapeutic opinions of one of the most influential personalities of the Parisian school.

In his first introductory lectures Bichat repeats his criticism, known from *General Anatomy,* and believes that the solution of the therapeutic puzzle will be brought about by an improved pathology. Today, he says, the same symptoms or the same organs are treated with the same medicaments, although one organ can suffer from different diseaes, which all need different methods of treatment. On the other hand, very different measures can have the same physiological effects.

Bichat said: "The subdivisions of materia medica have changed very often. The subdivisions are unavoidably very inadequate, especially with those medicaments that affect the whole organism. One must try to find out about the effects of a medicament. It is on this that one should base medical classifications and not on the scheme animal kingdom, vegetable kingdom, mineral kingdom, because it is of very minor importance whether a medicament belongs to one of these kingdoms." "One should study the effect of a medicament. If one does not know it, it is preferable to say nothing, instead of uttering hypotheses."

Bichat differentiates medicaments that influence the humors from those that affect the solid parts. The latter are the majority. He also differentiates between general and local effect. He begins in this lecture course an experimental examination of all therapeutic agents, e.g., drugs like laudanum, ipecacuanha, helleborus, ice, milk. Often he reports his own experiments with patients in the Hôtel Dieu. Death interrupted this research. The anatomy and pathology of tissues, as developed by Bichat, suggested the research for tissue-specific medicaments. It is difficult to decide where Bichat would have ended: as an empiricist, like Laennec or Louis, as an experimental pharmacologist, like Magendie, or as a "rational therapist," who based his rational therapeutics on insufficient pathological-physiological knowledge.

The latter way was the one followed by Bichat's admirer, Broussais, who in 1816 replaced Pinel as a leader of the Parisian school. Following this road, Broussais and his partisans did no small harm and failed eventually. Broussais reduced the whole of pathology to gastroenteritis. This gastroenteritis he treated with mucilaginous soups and extensive local application of leeches in the abdominal region. As far as medicaments are concerned, he ended paradoxically enough at the same practice as the one prescribed by his much maligned teacher Pinel. Only his theoretical explanation was different. He did not want to irritate the stomach. Broussais too practically did not give any drugs. He turned around Brunonianism. While Brown stimulated the too relaxed body, Broussais weakened the overstimulated body.

The murderous folly of Broussais' therapy is reflected in some figures: while France exported in 1820 still 1,158,000 leeches, France imported at the acme of Broussais' fame in 1833 no less than 41,654,300 leeches. Figures given by Lasègue and Regnauld in the *Archives générales* (January/February 1877) show that the abuse of leeches died down very slowly. The Hôtel Dieu in Paris in 1820 used 183,000 leeches per year. In 1836 the maximum of 1,280,000 was reached. But in 1850 still 316,000 were used. In 1870 eventually figures became smaller than in the time of Broussais and only 41,000 leeches were applied. Lasègue's data illustrate the slowness with which all forms of bleeding disappeared.

The third influential trend in the Parisian clinical school is represented by Corvisart, the body physician of Napoleon, and his pupils, Laennec, G. L. Bayle, etc. While we could call the attitude of Pinel an expectative skepticism and mild rationalism, that of Broussais an extreme rationalism and activism, Corvisart and his disciples exhibited a very characteristic mixture of skepticism, empiricism, and episodes of activism. It is typical for Corvisart that he praised as the greatest accomplishment of his friend and teacher Desbois de Rochefort the "épuration" (purge) of materia medica. Corvisart was in every respect an extreme skeptic. In his special field, the diseases of the heart, he bled and purged—he did not give digitalis! —but his opinion was that diseases of the heart can perhaps sometimes be prevented, but they can never be cured. The same point of view was accepted by his disciple Laennec. Typical for Corvisart is his aphorism: "Medicine is not the art to cure diseases; it is the art to treat them with the goal of cure, or to give the patient at least a feeling of well-being and to calm him."

G. L. Bayle, a disciple of Corvisart, says practically the same:

"Therapeutics is thus not in all cases the art of curing diseases, but the art of treating them decently." Bayle too was clearly a skeptic. That is why he logically had to put his hope into the healing power of nature. Of his seventeen "principles of therapeutics," no less than five underline the importance of the healing power of nature and of expectative therapeutics. He nevertheless gives numerous prescriptions following the old saying of Celsus: "It is better to try a medicament, the success of which is dubious, than to wait for certain death." In his own case—Bayle died early of pulmonary tuberculosis—he used no drugs whatsoever. He was clearly an empiricist. "If we would examine all diseases, we would see that we have no rational healing indication in most of them. Nevertheless some do exist which can be treated successfully with the specific or the empirical method, which is all the same in the end." For Bayle too the best hope for an improvement of therapeutics lays in better pathology. In his own special field, pulmonary tuberculosis, he is just as pessimistic as his teacher Corvisart was in his special field, the diseases of the heart. "Pulmonary tuberculosis is almost always incurable and fatal." He once says rather dryly that cases of tuberculosis or cancer that get cured have been diagnosed wrongly. Bayle, who gave much thought to therapeutics, saw very clearly the role of fashion in therapeutics. "Variations or modifications in the way of using indications depend entirely on the century in which one lives, on the country in which one practices, or—let us be frank about it—to a very large extent on fashion. There is nothing in the world that is not submitted to the whims of fashion, whether it be something very serious or something perfectly frivolous."

The therapeutic skepticism of the great Laennec is clearly revealed in his book on diseases of the chest. He turned down all the dear old methods that made life miserable for tuberculous patients, like bleeding, cantharides, softening medicaments, twenty-six other drugs, and all gases. The only curative agent in which the patriotic little Breton believed was "artificial sea air." It was at least harmless, and more agreeable than the simultaneously widely used cow-stable air therapeutics. He believed he had observed repeatedly nature curing phthisis. But medicine had not yet acquired the ability to achieve this result. In his lecture notes he reports over and over curative successes in certain cases, and attributes them always to the healing power of nature. Laennec examined his therapeutic results statistically.

It is all the more surprising that this skeptic empiricist suddenly took over the activistic treatment of pneumonia and articular rheumatism with high doses of tartar emetic, which had been introduced by Rasori whose theories he despised. The attacks of Broussais seem justified in this respect. Laennec proves here once more that even the greatest physicians are not always following logic when prescribing.

A very outspoken empiricist was Pierre Charles Alexandre Louis, who broke the influence of Broussais. Louis too wanted to derive therapeutics from therapeutics, an idea that Renouard preached as late as 1857. Before Louis, the hygienists Villermé and Parent Duchatelet and the clinicians Pinel, Esquirol, Rostan, G. L. Bayle, Laennec, Bouillaud, and Rayer had checked their therapeutic results with statistics. With Louis statistics, his numerical method, which the physicist Gavarret improved mathematically, became the central interest of research.

We can but agree with him if he states that only precise figures can pretend to validity, that data based exclusively on defective induction or only remembered facts can be but provisory, and that one should stop using terms like "often, rarely, many, etc." The new method was used particularly in the treatment of typhoid fever by Piedagnel and others, and of pneumonia by Grisolle, Dietl, and others.

In 1828, two years after his friend Marshall Hall, Louis, the skeptic, examined bleeding. He based his research on anatomically clearly defined diseases, like pneumonia, erysipelas, and angina. It is characteristic for his period that he did not dare to deal with the alternative "bleeding or no bleeding," but only with the alternative "much or little bleeding." His results were nevertheless sufficient to make this millenary, anemia-producing medical rite disappear slowly. In the seventies of the nineteenth century this became more visible. Purgatives and clysters, lacking just as much solid foundation and being made fun of as far back as Montaigne, survived into our own times.

It is no accident that the American disciples of Louis—Holmes, Bowditch, and Bartlett—left extremely skeptical statements on drugs.

Louis treated the same type of typhoid fever, against which Broussais mobilized regiments of leeches or Laennec gave large doses of tartar emetic, very simply with sufficient fluids, an ice bag on the head, and mild tonics. Similar treatments were given by Bretonneau and Rostan. The main merit of Louis is not contained in these details, but in the fact that he gave the clinically controlled experiment, which, next to the animal experiment, is the most important instrument to gain an objective therapeutic experience, a definite form. In this form the clinically controlled experiment spread into other countries.

The most important member of the last leading group of the classic Parisian school, the so-called eclectics, Gabriel Andral, has left us a slogan: "Better to give nothing than to give something doubtful." He did not think very highly of bleeding, but was more positively inclined toward purgatives and emetics. He oscillated between empiricism and rationalism. Another eclectic, the famous diagnostician Piorry, wrote a book on "the therapeutics of sound common sense." This book recommends primarily hygienic medication. Piorry was probably right in assuming that the great love of men for drugs is a form of superstition and laziness. It is much easier to take pills than to live hygienically. Trousseau criticized, on the one hand, those who were skeptical against the "classic," i.e., activistic, therapeutics. Fortunately he was simultaneously an admirer of the healing power of nature, which seemed to him proven through the successes of the homeopaths obtained in spite of the ineffectiveness of their remedies. Some of his therapeutic novelties (tracheotomy, paracentesis, cod liver oil) he inherited from his teacher Bretonneau.

In studying Bretonneau we can observe very well the increasing tendency toward local treatment. In the beginning Bretonneau had treated diphtheria as a general disease with mercury preparations. Later he treated diphtheria locally with hydrochloric acid, silver nitrate, and tracheotomy. Local treatment produces a trend toward surgical treatment, even with internal medicine specialists. The internist Récamier, who experimented with numerous forms of bathing and with many drugs, became an outstanding gynecological surgeon, and has to his credit the operative treatment of periuterine abscesses and retrouterine hematoma, the rediscovery of the speculum, the invention of the curette, and the first total extirpations of the cancerous uterus (after 1825). He also used drainage in empyema. Among the eclectics we still find terrible "vampires," like Bouillaud or Cruveilhier, otherwise so worthy of our admiration. Polypharmacy was for a while weakened in France, but advanced again around the middle of the century.

The other stronghold of therapeutic skepticism was Vienna which, since the middle of the eighteenth century, had become a great medical school. Skepticism was in Vienna a native product, as Erna Lesky has described so well. Its first protagonist was the Dutch obstetrician Johann Lukas Boer (1751–1835), who practiced after 1789 in Vienna and whose distrust of forceps and drugs was as great as was his trust in nature. The same point of view was defended by Johann Valentin von Hildenbrandt (1763–1818), who, from 1806, was professor of internal medicine. Suffering from typhoid fever in 1795, he had had such excellent experience in omitting all drugs that he now also wanted others to benefit from this method. His successor, von Raimann, followed the same line as did the professor of surgery, Kern (from 1823), who treated wounds only with water instead of devilish ointments.

Thus the Viennese skepticism would not have needed the Parisian stimulus, but it nevertheless strengthened this tendency in the so-called second Viennese school of Rokitansky, Skoda, Hebra, Semmelweis, etc. Skoda, a disciple of Raimann, was a therapeutic skeptic, but no more. Some younger members of the second Viennese school, like Joseph Dietl and Hamernik, developed therapeutic skepticism into therapeutic nihilism. But even with Dietl, nihilism was not a refusal of all drugs in principle. It was a refusal of contemporary drugs and methods, as they were scientifically without foundation, practically useless, if not harmful. Dietl expressed the hope that further scientific evolution of medicine would bring about a new scientific therapeutics. At the moment it was preferable to rely rather on the healing power of nature than on bleeding and the mess of useless or detrimental medicaments. Therapeutic nihilism could be no more than an episode. With Oppolzer therapeutics was again cultivated in Vienna. Leonardi stated in 1895 rightly that the advantages for medicine derived from the skepticism of the Viennese school were far greater than the often claimed disadvantages. Paris as well as Vienna became in this period a center of development of medical specialities, which have changed therapeutics considerably.

From France and Austria skepticism entered Germany and replaced the activism of Schoenlein. Eminent German clinicians like Oesterlen, Wunderlich, Kussmaul, Lebert, Ziemssen, and Nothnagel were very clearly therapeutic skeptics, and with Leyden and Strümpell the skeptic movement reaches into the twentieth century. As late as 1922, Strümpell differentiated necessary, useful, unnecessary, and harmful therapy. Another expression of a new critical spirit was the abolition of treatment by correspondence, as it had been practiced through centuries by all leaders of the profession. Treatment by correspondence survived only with sectarians.

A remark by G. F. Most in 1840 on "new" drugs between 1800 and 1840 illustrates how justifiable skepticism was: "Who now still prescribes tinctura cantharidum against whooping cough, in spite of Hufeland's praise of 1802? Who prescribes animal gelatin so highly recommended by Seguin in 1803 against intermittent fever? Who, following Husson, gratiola officinalis against gout? Who clematis erecta against rheumatism, scrofulosis and syphilis, which it cured in 1808? Who the bark of the tulip tree against malaria, as praised by von Hildenbrandt in 1809? Who tinctura antisyphilitica Bernardi of 1814? Who cortex tekornoque, curing pulmonary tuberculosis in 1814?"

The pragmatic physicians of Great Britain did not, during the first half of the nineteenth century, believe in theories, like the Germans, but they believed in drugs. All foreign observers were struck by the extensive use made of, for example, quinine or opium in England. Polypharmacy is prevalent in the English method of treating pulmonary tuberculosis. Fever was fought in the old energetic way by bleeding, emetics, purging, and fasting. Bloodletting had diminished since the times of Sydenham, but around 1800 the obituary notice of a Dublin lady reveals that during the last 10 years of her life she had suffered no less than 500 venesections.

Although British therapeutics was in general rather uniform, a milder tendency began to develop in the treatment of typhoid fever. This impressed the traveling Viennese professor Joseph Frank, who was surprised to find in Berlin that the very popular practitioner

Heim left this disease entirely to the healing power of nature. A milder treatment of fevers was favored by the famous Graves of Dublin, who wanted to have written on his tombstone: "He fed fevers."

Skepticism came relatively late to Great Britain and was primarily imported from France. All those mentioned in the following were either French trained or French influenced. Marshall Hall began in 1824 his attacks against the abuse of bloodletting, based on experiments. He too did not dare to attack bloodletting itself. Thus Hall was an important pioneer beyond the field of reflex studies. In 1857, J. H. Bennett of Edinburgh was more successful in his fight against bleeding. Around 1830 climatic therapy was taken up again by the later court physician James Clark. John Forbes, the translator of Laennec, criticized in 1845 energetically the prevailing polypharmacy and defended the healing power of nature, which he too saw proven by the successes of the homeopaths.

After the widespread iatrogenic alcoholism brought about by Brown and his disciples, the therapeutic role of alcohol was not mentioned very often during the first decades of the nineteenth century. In Meissner's *Encyklopädie der medizinischen Wissenschaften* (Leipzig, 1830), as well as in the *Dictionnaire de Médecine* (Trousseau, 1833; Jolly, 1835), alcohol is therapeutically recommended only for external use and as a solvent. The 1860s brought a new wave of enormous therapeutic use of alcohol. Now primarily acute fevers, caused by pneumonia, puerperal fever, or typhoid infection were treated with alcohol as a stimulus. Soon chronic fevers, too, for example, in pulmonary tuberculosis, were attacked with great quantities of cognac. This movement was led by the British anatomist Robert Bentley Todd (1809–1860), who, not too surprisingly, died early from "cirrhosis of liver and kidney." Todd's message was taken up by his disciple, F. A. Anstie (1833–1874), and spread rapidly in Great Britain as well as on the Continent. In France, Béhier was the main promoter of the new doctrine, in Germany Martins. It is significant that between 1860 and 1873 no less than fourteen doctoral theses were published in France praising this method of treatment. Doctoral theses are usually a faithful mirror of therapeutic fashions. Lasègue's statistics on the use of drugs in the Hôtel Dieu in Paris also reflect the extraordinary rise of therapeutic alcoholism between 1855 and 1876. In 1855 only 1270 liters of wine were given; in 1875 the quantity had risen to 37,578 liters.

Unfortunately, in the 1860s the so-called antipyretic wave (see below) started, and alcohol became an element of this kind of treatment. Consequently medical consumption of alcohol still increased. For Todd, alcohol had been above all a stimulant. For the partisans of the antipyretic wave, the internists, who based their actions on the experiments of C. Binz and his disciples, published after 1869, alcohol was chiefly a means to bring down the detrimental rise of temperature. Only toward the end of the century did this scientifically sanctioned form of alcoholism, often defended by intelligent and honest physicians, retreat thanks to the efforts of anti-alcoholic physicians like Forel, Bunge, and Bleuler.

The first half of the nineteenth century not only saw the bold attacks of skepticism in Paris, Vienna and other places; it saw another decisive turning point in the history of therapy, the turn from materia medica to pharmacology or, as we would like to call it, the turn toward physiologism. The main protagonists of this new therapeutics were the experimental physiologists and clinicians influenced by experimental physiology and experimental pathology. The old therapeutic art had slowly died in the long, painful chaos of the past 300 years. It was now slowly resurrected in the form of a science.

Some of the Parisian skeptics would perhaps have turned toward nihilism, like some Viennese men actually did. But this was prevented by a number of important chemical discoveries made in Paris and their application to medicine. This created new interest and confidence in drug treatment. Therewith a new era of therapeutics started, which was dominated by the newly created experimental pharmacology, which eliminated the old sterile opposition between "rational" and "empirical." Among the chemical discoveries the most important are the discoveries of several alkaloids which were most often made by the Parisian pharmacist Joseph Pelletier and his collaborators. We must not forget that Paris during this period was the world center not only of medicine but also of the sciences and especially chemistry; and chemistry was still to a large extent cultivated by pharmacists. Morphine had been discovered in 1805 by Sertürner. Pelletier discovered in 1817 (with Magendie) emetine, in 1818 (with Caventou) strychnine, in 1819 (with Caventou) brucine and veratrine, in 1820 (with Caventou) colchicine and quinine. P. J. Robiquet discovered in 1821 caffeine and in 1832 codeine. In the same years the halogens (iodine, bromine, chlorine, etc.) were discovered and introduced in medicine. For the first time in history clinicians and physiologists had at their disposal a whole series of chemically pure and known substances of vegetable origin which could always be used in the same quantity. Former extracts and raw products had oscillated continuously in their contents of active substance. The well-known chemist Chevreul (1786–1889) saw clearly this historical turning point.

It is a paradox that this renaissance of drug therapy and general treatment and the creation of a new science, experimental pharmacology, were brought about by the most skeptical of all Paris clinicians, the physiologist Magendie.

Magendie was born in 1783, the son of a surgeon and democrat in Bordeaux. He died in Paris in 1855. All his life long he made a living as a practicing physician and became famous in this respect, as is obvious from the fact that Balzac makes him one of the three great consultants of the period in his *Peau de chagrin;* the others are Broussais and Récamier. His fame as practicing physician increased very much through the fact that in 1818 he obtained an official position at the Hôtel Dieu. But his heart belonged to science. From 1808 he experimented and published in the fields of physiology, pathology, and pharmacology, and is therewith the initiator of modern experimental physiology, pathology, and pharmacology. In 1821 he became a member of the Academy of Sciences, and in 1822 he published his most famous physiological discovery, the so-called Bell law of the motor function of the anterior and the sensory function of the posterior roots of the spinal marrow. External recognition of his scientific accomplishments came late and outside of the faculty; in 1830 Magendie became professor at the Collège de France. Magendie was also very active in public health.

Magendie was the most radical adversary of bloodletting in the Parisian school. He strictly prohibited his interns to bleed. In a discussion in the Academy of Medicine concerning the value of bleeding he stated that his patients recovered without being bled. He was somewhat surprised when his colleagues reacted in gay laughter. Like the proverbial husband, he was the only one who did not know that his interns were so firmly convinced of the lifesaving function of bleeding that they did not dare, in the interest of their patients, to obey the orders of their chief and bled secretly. This shows that at that time bloodletting must have held in France, and not only in France, a truly divine position. Otherwise such an act of disobedience would be unthinkable.

Magendie's formulary (*Formulaire pour la préparation et l'emploi de plusieurs nouveaux médicaments*) appeared for the first time in Paris in 1821. One edition followed the other. We use below primarily the eighth, of 1835. Although others, like Barbier in the second edition of his treatise of materia medica (1824) and Julia Fontenelle (*Archives générales,* volume IV [1824], 152), rapidly followed Magendie along this road, the *Formulaire* remains the basic document of the new experimental-pharmacological trend.

Magendie explains in his preface that his work is based on the eventual discovery of chemically pure drugs and on the disappearance of the old prejudice that drugs and poisons have a basically different effect in men and in animals.

In 1809 Magendie had experimentally demonstrated the influence of nux vomica on the spinal marrow. It is therefore not surprising that the first medicament of his *Formulaire* is strychnine. As for all the following substances he discusses for strychnine the following points: preparation from raw materials, physical and chemical properties, effect in the animal, effect in the healthy and sick man, indication, form of application (prescriptions for pills, tinctures, the different salts of the substance). In the same way he discusses brucine, morphine, narcotine, narceine, meconine and codeine, which as a hypnotic he judges superior to morphine. The next substances discussed are emetine (discovered by him in collaboration with Pelletier in 1817), veratrine, the alkaloids of the Peruvian bark: quinine and cinchonine. Together with Double, Villermé, and Chomel he had introduced these alkaloids in practical medicine against considerable resistance. Magendie was not afraid of recommending, since 1817, prussic acid—it is true in small doses —as a cough mixture, but he warned against the dangers of the substance.

Iodine, discovered in 1811 by Courtois, was, according to Magendie, used widely against goiter on the recommendation of Coindet of Geneva (1819). As goiter and scrofulosis have been confused continuously, it is not surprising that it was also used in scrofulosis. Richond had given it successfully against syphilis in 1824. It was furthermore thought to be a strong emmenagogue. Magendie reports the use of iodine in tuberculosis, cancer, and epilepsy. He regards bromine (discovered in 1826 by Balard) as an equivalent of iodine. Chlorine (discovered by Scheele in 1774), he used primarily for disinfection, also in wounds and against pulmonary diseases.

Solanine, delphinine, gentianine, and lupuline had been tested in animal experiments, but no therapeutic application for them had been found. Oil of croton is a drastic; given intravenously in the animal experiment, it kills.* Segalas had discovered the diuretic effect of urea in the intravenous animal experiment. Thridace or the juice of lettuce is, according to François, a sedative, and reduces the body temperature and the pulse rate.

The salts of gold which were given in syphilis and scrofulosis were very toxic in the intravenous animal experiments of the famous toxicologist Orfila. Grenadine and fern are proven remedies against intestinal worms. Magendie is very reserved concerning the marvellous results of others with phosphorus. But he sees clearly that the discovery of this substance in the brain by Couerbe will bring about a new fashion of its therapeutic application.

Sodium and potassium bicarbonate had been used since Darcet (1826) in gastric hyperacidity. Magendie feels that the digitalin of the Geneva pharmacist Auguste Leroy, who also did interesting animal experiments with this substance, has still to be tested more thoroughly. Salicin, which he uses against fever, is no alkaloid. In dyspepsia he gives lactic acid.

These are the new drugs of the Parisian school that either replaced or complemented the traditional preparations of vegetable or mineral (antimony, arsenic, mercury) origin.

---

* Intravenous medication had been used long before Magendie (see H. Buess, *CIBA Zeitschrift* No. 100, March 1946). In France, Percy and Ch. N. Laurent had introduced in 1797 the intravenous treatment of tetanus by opium. But the use of the intravenous method by Magendie in the animal experiment, as well as in his treatment of rabies, drew undoubtedly more attention to the method. It was widely used only in the last quarter of the nineteenth century. Subcutaneous injections were introduced by Rynd (1844) and Alexander Wood (1853).

The most important contributions of Magendie are not single discoveries, but the introduction of a new scientific principle, which made it possible to replace "systems" by objective experiments and discussions, and to eliminate the old sterile opposition of "rationalism" and "empiricism." Germany was at that time scientifically still so underdeveloped that a respected author like G. A. Richter could claim in 1826 that animal experiments were irrelevant for therapeutics and that "living" chemistry had nothing to do with "dead" chemistry.

The work of Magendie was continued in France in the most brilliant way by his disciple, the physiologist Claude Bernard. Bernard, by the way, was no longer a practitioner, but showed sympathies for the healing power of nature and neural pathology. The new pharmacology was soon (see below) to be very successful in Germany, Austria, and Great Britain. The self-experiments of J. E. Purkinjé (1787–1869) deserve honorable mention in these early pharmacological efforts.

As we have seen, at the turn of the nineteenth century a whole series of effective drugs entered the therapeutic scene. Unfortunately they were used in a rather discreditable way. This can be very easily documented by perusal of the anthology of Antoine L. Bayle (the nephew of Gaspard L. Bayle), *Bibliothèque thérapeutique,* published in 1828. This misuse occurred at a time when, in view of the general evolution of medicine and the sciences, one was entitled to hope for better results. Unfortunately the psychological mechanisms that were manifest then are still observable today. I would like to support this claim by a short examination of the history of digitalis, iodine, and quinine.

Withering had discovered digitalis in 1785 as a diuretic affecting the heart. Within the next twenty years digitalis was transformed into a panacea. As early as 1799 it was regarded as extremely successful against tuberculosis (Ferriar, G. L. Bayle). For Hufeland, it was the remedy against scrofulosis; Quarin was of the same opinion. Pneumonia, typhoid fever, and many other diseases were "successfully" treated with digitalis. Digitalis "cured" also mental disease, although it is now known that it can produce depressions. Relatively reserved were the French skeptics around 1830, but even they were submerged by a new wave of polypharmacy. In spite of basing his recommendations in general on thorough experimental research, the famous Berlin clinician, the experimental pathologist Ludwig Traube, recommended in the 1860s digitalis in pneumonia, a recommendation that was followed by some into the twentieth century. Only in the 1890s did digitalis become again what it actually was: a specific in certain heart diseases!

Iodine had a very similar fate. Coindet had recommended it in 1819 for the treatment of goiter. But he himself was not able to resist the temptation to use the new substance as a panacea, and recommended it in scrofulosis. This is not so surprising, in view of the fact that goiter and scrofulosis were very often confused at that time. Coindet found iodine also successful in dysmenorrhea, chlorosis, and syphilis. Iodine became soon very prominent in the treatment of syphilis. In this field, gold, which for centuries had been promoted to do the possible and the impossible, had just proven again to be very disappointing. Within ten years iodine became also a remedy for cancer, different skin diseases, heart diseases, epilepsy, tuberculosis, malaria, cholera and arteriosclerosis. Only in the middle of our own century has the use of iodine been limited to the treatment of thyroid gland diseases and use as an external antiseptic.

Peruvian bark had been for a long time a panacea. When, in 1820, quinine was isolated from the bark, the new alkaloid also was used as a panacea. In spite of all the evidence that it was a specific for malaria, quinine was given against all fevers. As a matter of fact, in the one fever for which it was specific, it appeared most of the time only in fourth place of possible treatments after emetics, cathartics, and venesection. It was regarded as a sovereign remedy in the case of neuralgia or cachexy. It had supposedly a double effect: antifebrile and as a tonic. Quinine too was used in a more rational way only in the 1890s. All three medicaments were given in far too high doses very often.

Under these circumstances, it is not surprising that the new remedies could not solve the problems of therapeutics for the time being. Essential testing methods (animal experiment, clinically controlled experiments, statistics) were known, but were not used often enough and were not used in a really competent and precise fashion. Only better knowledge of the pathophysiology of so-called dropsy, of goiter, of malaria, brought about a more rational use of these panaceas.

XI

Middle of the
Nineteenth Century:
The Acme of the Chaos, Sects,
Errors of Pharmacology, Synthetic
Drugs

AROUND THE middle of the nineteenth century the therapeutic chaos reached its acme. On March 12, 1851, the Leipzig clinician C. A. Wunderlich said in his introductory lecture: "There was once a time, and it is not so long ago, when the expression to treat a patient according to the rules of the art, lege artis, had a sense. In the old time, different medical schools and sects did exist simultaneously or successively. They fought each other's theories and therapeutic principles. But within the school there existed firm rules. The choice of the method of treatment was not given to the will of the individual. Today, instead of doctrinary rigidity, we encounter the most complete therapeutic anarchy." The old humoralist tendency with its evacuating therapeutics did still exist in the background. Leading clinicians of the period, like Schoenlein, Lebert, Lasègue, were in spite of Louis and Marshall Hall still "vampirists." In 1838 Junod still invented a cupping shoe. In 1862 the rather sensible Freiburg clinician Baumgärtner regarded as the five pillars of therapeutics: bloodletting, emetics, purgatives, opium, quinine. Then came calomel, chloroform, potassium iodide, iron, digitalis, cod liver oil, and wine. Eventually heat, cold, water, and diet were quoted. In the 1870s dissertations were still published in Munich which praised derivation, and the famous Parisian hematologist Hayem preached as late as 1887 revulsion and derivation.

In spite of all skeptical trends in Paris, in Vienna, and even in Germany (Wunderlich said once: "There are no diseases that could not be cured without so-called drugs"), polypharmacy was still indescribable. Fechner mocked this situation in saying: "Really a friend of mankind must be most happy when regarding our materia medica and seeing that it shows the most certain signs that our present medicine will soon reach the peak of its progress, if it has not reached it already. The ancients were glad to have one drug against each disease, and against many they did not have any. How much happier are we! We do not only have at our disposal innumerable drugs against each single disease, but each single remedy cures now innumerable diseases. The triumph of science is characterized by the fact that now we have against the most incurable diseases the most numerous and the most effective drugs. Therefore if somebody, after reading a book on materia medica, is left the choice whether he would much rather have a head cold or pulmonary tuberculosis, he will, if he has only a modest measure of common sense, certainly choose the latter. We possess so excellent and so numerous drugs against it, that if somebody would have coughed up already half of his lung, the other half would become so clean and healthy with our drugs that it can replace the function of the lost half. Epilepsy, rabies and other things of this kind are now only jokes, because every day we discover new drugs against them, and, as far as I remember, exclusively infallible ones."

It is typical for the abuse of calomel, mostly based on humoralism, that the German anatomists entertained in the 1850s a spirited discussion on whether mercury was a normal constituent of the human bone or not. In many anatomical institutes no mercury-free bones were found.

One shudders in reading how cholera was handled during the great epidemics of the nineteenth century by most physicians. Charles Rosenberg reports in his *Cholera Years* (Chicago, 1962) that calomel was combined with laudanum, pepper, jalap, sulfur, tobacco clyster, electrization, strychnine, aconite, or morphine. This in spite of the fact that Latta recommended in Edinburgh as early as 1832 the injection of saline solutions, which is still practiced. He did not find many followers at that time. K. G. Neumann was undoubtedly right when he assumed that it was not scrofulosis, but the intensive methods of treatment with antimony, leeches, and mercury that killed so many children. By a hair's breadth mankind escaped "syphilization," i.e., the preventive inoculation of syphilis, which had been developed as a parallel to smallpox vaccination. "Only" several hundred people were vaccinated with syphilis. Under these circumstances it is not surprising that Lasègue's opinion on the therapeutic literature of this time is not exactly flattering: "Original publications are only in exceptional cases disinterested. Either the authors have become victims of hasty convictions, or they have been inspired by less excusable sentiments." Alex Berman established in 1954 a very impressive balance sheet of the so-called heroic methods in therapeutics. James Marion Sims, the great American gynecological surgeon, says in his memoirs in his short, honest and forthright manner: "Practice of that time (around 1840) was heroic. It was murderous. I did not know anything of medicine, but I had enough common sense to see that physicians killed their patients, that medicine was no

exact science, that it proceeded empirically and that it was preferable to put one's confidence into nature, and not in the dangerous
skill of physicians."

Skepticism and the new pharmacology appealed only to an elite.
To the mass of the bewildered they offered little consolation. It is
therefore not surprising that many people abandoned official medicine and followed the so-called sects. Medicine suffered a great
crisis of confidence. Not only the application of the remedies but
the remedies themselves were now questioned. We have mentioned
already the homeopaths as profiting from this crisis. Then came
the hydropaths. Water had an honorable past in Babylonian, Jewish, Hippocratic medicine and with Asklepiades and Galen. Floyer
and Currie had resurrected its therapeutic use in the eighteenth century. Now water produced miracles in the hands of a Silesian peasant called Priessnitz (1799–1851) and the Bavarian clergyman
Kneipp. They inundated their patients externally and internally. Another peasant, Schroth, dried them out. It helped too. The special
diets of a Banting or Graham became very popular. The reform of
Hahnemann consisted in a new application of traditional remedies.
Other so-called biochemical sects grew out of his sect. The so-called
medicine of experience of Rademacher as well as the nature medicine of a Felke attracted many patients.

The young United States developed her own sects, like the osteo-
paths (1874), the chiropractitioners (1855), and Christian Scientists (around 1860), which now invaded Europe. Everywhere the
spiritualists were active as therapeutic sectarians. The French scientist and statesman Raspail developed his own "system," which recommended a harmless panacea (camphor) and, twenty years before
Pasteur and thirty years before Lister, prevention against micro-
scopic disease-producing organisms and clean instruments. It is characteristic of the crisis of confidence that Raspail did not want to
have an official M.D., because he was afraid that this would deprive
him of the confidence of his proletarian patients!

Under the pressure of these mass movements and out of its own
therapeutic skepticism, official medicine opened its door to the so-
called natural methods. Water, for example, was introduced by Vog-
ler, Braun, Brandt, and others, partly as an antipyretic, into official
therapeutics. Niemeyer preached fresh air. A special application of

climatotherapy was the first effective treatment of pulmonary tuberculosis by air cures, inaugurated by Brehmer in Gerbersdorf in
1854. Laymen like Jahn and Lingg promoted gymnastics. Lingg's
resurrecting of massage was particularly meritorious. Orthodox
medical men decided under the influence of these movements to
teach healthful behavior to the masses as a prophylactic. Diet was
again put into practice. The revival of physical therapy did not occur
without regrettable errors, like the "suspension method" to cure
tabes which was no less regrettable than the later "surgery of tabes."
Internal reforms thus slowly reestablished the credit of official medicine. It increased tremendously, thanks to the steep progress of
surgery after the middle of the century, which followed the invention of anesthesia and antisepsis-asepsis.

Another minority in therapeutics were the "physiologists." Although counting several leaders of the profession in their ranks, they
never gained mass influence. They believed in practicing rationally
on the basis of experimental physiology and experimental pharmacology. They gave more attention to general treatment. Some of
them, like Wunderlich, proceeded for a while with much arrogance.
Yet disappointed by his "rational" therapeutics, Wunderlich re-
treated to the Parisian statistical empiricism of his youth.

Progress in pharmacology was and could be only very slow.
France had brilliant representatives of this new discipline, like Magendie and Claude Bernard. It was well known that they had to
work outside of the medical faculties dominated by pure clinicians.
Therefore pharmacology found its full academic recognition only in
the German language era. This is above all the work of R. Buchheim
(1820–1879), a disciple of E. H. Weber, who worked from 1846
to 1867 in Dorpat and founded there with his private means the
first pharmacological institute. His disciple, O. Schmiedeberg (1838–
1921), was after 1872 professor in Strasbourg. He was an enor-
mously influential teacher. Supposedly his disciples have filled forty
chairs in ten countries. He is well known for his work on digitalis
and histamine. Another important pharmacological center was the
Vienna institute created by Karl Damian Ritter von Schroff (1802–
1887). Edinburgh was, through the efforts of Sir Robert Christison
(1797–1882), the third early pharmacological research center after
Paris and Dorpat. The Edinburgh tradition was continued ably

through Christison's disciples, Benjamin Ward Richardson, Alexander Crum Brown, and Thomas Frazer, who tried, from the beginning of the 1860s, to study the connection between chemical constitution and pharmacological effect. Thomas Lauder Brunton became famous through the introduction of amyl nitrate in angina pectoris (1867). His textbook of pharmacology of 1885 became the international leader.

Cellular theory and cellular pathology spread rapidly around the middle of the nineteenth century. It is very interesting and significant that no cellular therapy developed during this period. The protagonists of cellular theory and cellular pathology, like Virchow, Lebert, and Remak, were therapeutically only disciples of Schoenlein, who became more skeptical in the course of the years. They did not give the world a cellular therapy. Neither did those clinicians who were disciples of Virchow and had strong therapeutic interests, like Leyden, Ziemssen, and Nothnagel. Attempts to create a cellular therapy, like those of F. A. Hoffmann, H. Schultz, or Louis Lewin, were unsuccessful. Only fifty years after the introduction of cellular pathology did Paul Ehrlich develop theoretically and practically a therapy derived from the Virchowian idea of the affinity of cell and drug, and which therefore deserves the name of cellular therapy.

The progress of physiologism, of experimental pharmacology, was slow as it depended on the progress of chemistry and physics. Besides, the first steps of physiologism were not free from errors. We have seen this in the case of iodine and quinine. The greatest and most influential mistake of physiologism is the so-called antipyretic wave, which started in the 1860s and came to an end only at the beginning of the twentieth century. It grew out of the scientific occupation with fever. Systematic measurement of temperature of different French (Gavarret, Récamier, Andral) and German (Bärensprung, Traube) clinicians culminated in the book of Wunderlich of 1868 on body temperature. Wunderlich's curves were extremely suggestive. Simultaneously Liebermeister, the great promoter of the antipyretic wave, demonstrated that during fever the body uses more of its substance than normally. This seemed to prove the detrimental nature of fever, which had been regarded so long as a useful reaction of nature. The clinicians, tired of expectation, saw here the scientific basis for a new active method to reduce temperature, antipyresis.

Thus Briquet, Traube, and Liebermeister started at the end of the 1860s to act antipyretically. In the beginning they used the traditional antipyretic means, like cold water, digitalis, quinine, and veratrine, to reduce fever. When in 1871 C. E. Buss introduced the clinical use of salicylic acid, the chemical industry started to bring to the market continuously new and better adapted antipyretic substances, which it advertised heavily. This strengthened, of course, the antipyretic movement considerably.

The first synthetic drugs of the chemical industry owe, like many of their successors, their existence to the relationship between dyes and drugs. The English chemist W. H. Perkin examined in the 1850s tar waste products in order to produce drugs (carbolic acid was another tar waste product). Perkin was particularly interested in a drug to replace quinine. For the time being all he discovered was a whole series of important dyes. It was only later that dyes became again medicaments, such as trypan red and the sulfonamides.

The first synthetic drug to play a medical role was salicylic acid, synthesized by Kolbe in 1874 (salicylic acid had been extracted as early as 1838 out of salicin, and its constitution had been cleared up in 1853). Buss introduced it into therapeutics in 1875 against poly-arthritis. He was followed by Sticker (1876) and G. Sée (1877). Soon salicylic acid became above all an antipyretic drug and a panacea, even outside of military circles.

The next popular synthetic drug was antipyrine, found by Knorr in 1884, when looking for a replacement for quinine. The tempera-ture-reducing effect of antipyrine was discovered by Filhene in 1884. Then followed sulfonal (Baumann, 1886), antifebrin (Cahn-Hepp, 1887), phenacetin (Hinsberg and Kant, 1887). All these medica-ments were supposed to be specifics and rationally applied, as the harmfulness of fever had now become a dogma. The antipyretics became panaceas. Only extended experience with this way of treat-ing fevers, better insight into the nature of fever, and above all the discovery of curative effects of fever in certain diseases brought about a change. It was realized that the above-mentioned synthetic drugs had had primarily a symptomatic action. Through the gen-eralization of the cases, where fever was curative, the antipyretic wave was replaced now by a no less irrational "pyretic wave." The old saying of George Wedekind (1791) is unfortunately still valid:

"Even a superficial study of the history of medicine reveals how easily the great mass of physicians always fell from one extreme into the other, how small always the number of the sages was who acted on the basis of reasons which they had thought about themselves, and who therefore applied the *medium tenere beati* (happy those who stick to the middle of the road)." Needless to say that this quality of physicians, to depend on fashion, is but a generalized human trend.

In the case of the synthetic hypnotics—chloral hydrate (Oskar Liebreich, 1869), paraldehyde (1884), veronal (Emil Fischer, 1903)—it was clear from the very beginning that they had only a symptomatic effect. In February 1879, W. F. Loebisch and Prokop von Rokitansky published under the editorship of Professor Dr. Johannes Schnitzler a survey of newer drugs, their indications and effects. The list of the drugs discussed in this little monograph illustrates very well the tendencies of the period in drug therapy. Loebisch and Rokitansky, junior, discussed and recommended amyl nitrate, pilocarpine, pancreatin, apomorphine, salicylic acid, chloral hydrate, and trimethylamine. Today, ninety years later, some of these medicaments are still used.

The synthetic drugs brought to an end a whole era of therapeutics, the era of herbs. Chemical industry now became a most influential partner of therapy. The industrial production of drugs had begun before the second half of the nineteenth century. Monasteries and large pharmacies had been engaged for centuries in the mass production of proprietary medicines. Modern industrial production of drugs starts after the discovery of the alkaloids. A particularly strong need for quinine existed at a time when malaria was very widespread even in Europe. Some pharmacists started now with the industrial production of alkaloids, e.g., the pharmacist Merck in Darmstadt around 1826, the pharmacist Schering around 1855, and the pharmacist Nestlé in 1865. The same evolution was observable among French, American, and British apothecaries. The next object of mass production was the anesthetics. These were no longer plant products, but pure chemicals. Pharmacology became more and more chemical. Part of the pharmaceutical industry grew out of the large-scale trade with chemicals (Boehringer).

Another part of the pharmaceutical industry had very different roots. It was a child of the dye industry, which had developed from the processing of tar products. This dye industry, which later became to a large extent pharmaceutical, had not accidentally developed in regions with textile industry; e.g., the firm of Bayer was founded in 1863 in Wuppertal. The Hoechst factories, founded in 1863 as dye factories, produced in 1883 the first quinine ersatz. Bayer opened its pharmaceutical activities in 1886 with phenacetin. The pharmaceutical-chemical industry synthesizes today not only chemicals but also alkaloids, hormones, vitamins, and antibiotics, which originally were products of nature. Pharmaceutical industry is as profitable as it is important and useful. Its attempts to present itself to the public as a purely philanthropic or scientific enterprise are sometimes rather annoying. In the United States, pharmaceutical industry spends twice as much for advertising as for research and invests for advertising ten times as much out of its income as the automobile industry and twice as much as the tobacco and liquor industries. For other countries no data are available. They would probably be very similar. The pharmaceutical industry would, of course, never spend such sums for advertising if it could not assume that even physicians are very easily influenced in this way.

Winfried Schroeder in 1960 published an excellent monograph, *Die pharmazeutisch-chemischen Produkte deutscher Apotheken zu Beginn des naturwissenschaftlich-industriellen Zeitalters,* wherein he uses the methods developed by Wolfgang Schneider, which had previously yielded such excellent results in the monograph of Gerald Schroeder (see our chapter on the seventeenth century). Winfried Schroeder shows that the total number of official medical substances decreased because certain combination preparations and chemically impure inorganic chemicals disappeared from the pharmacopoeias. Organic chemical products (natural substances like morphine, quinine, picrotoxin) increased. Industry was able to produce them not only cheaper but also purer than the pharmacists could.

XII

End of the Nineteenth Century: The Breakthrough to Modern Therapeutics by Way of Serum Therapy. Psychotherapeutic and Psychosomatic Endeavors

THE RESULTS of clinical and pathological research cumulating since the beginning of the nineteenth century, the results of Pinel, Laennec, Graves, Bright, Skoda, Rokitansky, Virchow, Kussmaul, Charcot, Gowers, etc., had made the nineteenth century a century of pathology. Bacteriology, flourishing during the second half of the century, had brought more than some important vaccinations. It had stimulated hygiene to such an extent that one can speak of an era of public health, following the era of pathology. It is primarily public health that produced the dramatic increase of average life expectation during the twentieth century. Surgery too owed to bacteriology asepsis and therewith its sudden progress. But the rest of therapeutics lagged still behind in spite of important pharmacological results, in spite of valuable synthetic products. Only at the end of the century did the breakthrough occur that has made it possible to claim that the new era in medicine, beginning in the 1930s, is an era of therapeutics.

This important and decisive turning point in the development of therapeutics was not brought about by synthetic products, but by natural products, the curative sera. For decades the bacteriological laboratory had made possible enormous successes in surgery and preventive medicine. Now it became also the root of the great new therapeutic successes by way of medicaments. The specific causative agents, discovered by bacteriology, suggested a search for specific remedies. In 1862 the then 76-year-old chemist Chevreul had a clear foreboding of this situation when he wrote: "We must exploit the fact that one is able to neutralize chemically certain qualities, while others continue to exist. We will find means to neutralize the microorganisms." Lasègue too assumed in 1876: "Perhaps the time is near when, instead of only studying the sequence of disease, we will try to find the causes." This old dream of causal treatment, of the specific and etiological remedy, now became reality for the first time through serum therapy. An era that had lasted for several millennia, an era of almost exclusively symptomatic treatment in internal medicine, came to an end. It was a turning point that was recognized as such by the contemporaries.

King had talked in 1693 of disinfection in diseases. Pringle had made in vitro experiments with quinine and paramecia. Hill, Vriesberg, Needham, Spallanzani, and others had made similar attempts.

After the discovery of pathogenic microorganisms by Davaine, Pasteur, Koch, and others, and after Lister's great successes with external disinfection, Koch and Chamberland had tried the so-called internal disinfection. Koch had looked for specific substances against specific pathogenic microorganisms. The young military physician E. Behring had followed him along this road; but his experiments, like all similar experiments, had shown the traditional disinfectants to be too toxic. Behring asked himself whether disinfectants could perhaps be found in nature. The Wiesbaden Congress for internal medicine of 1883 had just turned down emphatically such an assumption. But there remained, for example, the strange fact that the serum of rats could kill anthrax bacilli. The discoveries of Roux and Yersin in 1888 and of Faber and Kitasato in 1890—that in diphtheria or tetanus, it is not the bacillus that damages, but its toxins—brought Behring one step further forward. He was also strongly influenced by the experiments of Ehrlich with ricine, abrine, and other poisonous substances with which Ehrlich was able to produce immunity. Perhaps therapeutics should aim at the toxins.

In 1890 Behring was able to demonstrate that in the serum of guinea pigs infected with diphtheria, antitoxins are formed. In 1893 he began to produce an antidiphtheria serum which was standardized with the help of Ehrlich. In 1901 Behring deservedly received the first medical Nobel Prize. The discovery of Behring's was of tremendous practical usefulness and importance in treating such dangerous bacterial infections as diphtheria and later many others, amongst them pneumonia. In tetanus and snakebite these sera are still used. This was before the era of chemotherapy and antibiotics. But the practical importance of the discovery was overshadowed by its basic meaning. It was now proven that it was possible to fight infections with specific substances, which attack the cause of the infection and which had been found in the laboratory. This success of, what Ehrlich called, passive immunization revived activities in the field of active immunizations, of vaccinations, which had been started by Jenner and Pasteur. During the 1890s vaccinations against typhoid fever, cholera and plague were developed. The treatment with gamma globulin is a later form of therapy.

Another group of curative substances, produced by nature, and found toward the end of the nineteenth century in the laboratories, were the hormones. Hormone therapy began very dramatically in 1889 through the self-treatment of the famous Parisian physiologist Charles Edouard Brown-Séquard with testicular extracts. It rejuvenated him so rapidly that within two weeks he lost his constipation, but acquired in exchange whooping cough. Although the objective value of these experiments is doubtful, they nevertheless opened up the field of internal secretion and of the treatment with extracts of hormone-producing glands. In 1891 Murray was able to cure myxedema with thyroid extracts.

The fact that psychological factors play a great role in the genesis as well as in the therapeutics of diseases has never escaped physicians who were good observers. We have drawn attention to this in our treatment of Greek, Roman, Western medieval, Arabic, Hindu, Renaissance, seventeenth- and eighteenth-century medicine. This fact is generally recognized but is denied in certain quarters for the second half of the nineteenth century, against which it is fashionable to-day to develop oedipal prejudices. It seems therefore necessary to have a look at the facts instead of deciding the matter on the basis of the preconceived opinion that the "materialistic nineteenth century" could not have had psychosomatic insights. My short survey is very far from being complete; I am only discussing the psychosomatics of the specialists in internal medicine, and even among those I have to limit myself to the two most important clinical schools of the nineteenth century: the French and the German.

The leading clinical school of the first half of the nineteenth century was the French. It is undeniable that its main interest centered in the fields of pathological anatomy and physical diagnosis. But as these French clinicians were complete human beings, and not diagnostic computers, they were of course interested in all aspects of disease, including the psychological ones, which they often called "moral." They were all the more interested in psychological aspects as they were skeptical concerning traditional therapeutics and welcomed warmly psychotherapeutic additions to their therapeutic armamentarium. The philosophical precursor of the Parisian school, Cabanis, produced in his *Relations between the Physical and the Moral in Men* the classic on psychosomatic relations, demonstrated clearly the disease-producing influence of "moral" elements, and asked for psychotherapeutics. It is not surprising that we find in the writings of Pinel, a friend of Cabanis and the first leading clinician of the school, now remembered mostly as a psychiatrist, numerous psychosomatic passages. He was familiar with the neuroses of the gastrointestinal tract, the heart, and hearing. Some of what he, like many other contemporaries, writes could be even called a kind of hyperpsychosomatism. He believed, for example, in psychological commotion as a cause of erysipelas, gout, and epilepsy. He asked for moral treatment, especially in the case of hypochondria that was characterized by colic, vomiting, spasms, anxiety, melancholia, and confusion. The tradition of Cabanis lasted through Alibert, Moreau, Cérise, Bouchut, etc., to Charcot. Moral treatment is described, for example, in Cruveilhier, Rayer, Alibert, Véron, and Lachaise. Even the bloodthirsty disciple and adversary of Pinel, Broussais, who had reduced all diseases to gastroenteritis, and all therapeutics to leeches, knew that a gastroenteritis can have psychological sources. Bouillaud, a disciple of Broussais, was very familiar with the neurosis of the heart with palpitations, syncope, etc., and recommended psychotherapy.

The great Corvisart mentions right at the beginning of his famous work on the diseases of the heart the great influence of the psyche on the heart. In his translation of Auenbrugger's book on percussion, which consists 70 percent of his own additions, we find descriptions of psychosomatic syndromes like the so-called jealousy of children. Gaspard Laurent Bayle, the disciple of Corvisart, recommended strongly the study of psychology for the physician. Bayle knew that psychic phenomena could be the cause as well as the effect of disease. He describes two "psychosomatic" cases of death, but warns against a hyperpsychosomatism, which, for example, explains cancer of the stomach by emotions.

This hyperpsychosomatic point of view was defended by Théophile Laennec, the friend of Bayle's and the most important disciple of Corvisart. Laennec also believed that psychological causes were the only firmly established causes of pulmonary tuberculosis. Laennec insisted on the existence of neurosis as a functional disease, independent of pathological-anatomical changes. Such neuroses were to him, for example, asthma or palpitations.

Pierre Charles Alexandre Louis is the only one of the great Parisian clinicians who has not left any psychosomatic discussions in print. His friend Chomel, however, attributed a large part of the cases of typhoid fever to nostalgia. Chomel became, in later stages of his career, more and more aware of the psychosomatic element in so-called dyspepsia. He collected these observations in private practice, which in general is more suited for psychosomatic observations than the assembly lines of large hospitals. In general with all these clinicians, psychosomatic insight increased with growing experience. Grisolle, a disciple of Chomel, was very interested in psychosomatics. Piorry, the master of percussion, was skeptical in relation to psychosomatic explanations of typhoid fever, but knew very well the psychosomatic element in heart disease, and above all in impotence, which he successfully treated by psychotherapy. The famous Andral was another believer in the emotional roots of cancer of the stomach. In general he believed that functional disturbances could change into organic lesions. Cruveilhier described the psychological elements in ulcer of the stomach. Trousseau, the last famous representative of the Parisian school, described under the heading of neurosis: diarrhea, dyspepsia, enuresis, hyperthyroidism, angina pectoris, and asthma. He was himself a sufferer from asthma and has left us a classic description of an attack, caused by intense emotion. He observed that one of these neuroses could be replaced by another. Not only medical books in France are very rich in psychosomatic data during this period; literary fiction overflows with them.

During the second half of the nineteenth century the German clinicians became international leaders. It is understandable that these clinicians were skeptical and prosaic. They had just survived a thirty-year flood of Romantic blah-blah, which had completely paralyzed German medicine. The first famous German clinician, Johann Lukas Schoenlein, was still a Romantic in Würzburg, but introduced French diagnostics into the German clinics in Zurich and Berlin. In his written lectures not much concerning psychological causes of disease or psychotherapy can be found. But according to the testimony of his disciple, Leyden, Schoenlein was convinced that, in the field of cardiac disease, psychogenesis was possible and psychotherapy could be valuable. The Leipzig clinician Wunderlich, who introduced routine thermometry, knew psychological causes in heart diseases, gastric ulcer, liver diseases, anemia, and apoplexy. The clinician H. Lebert, better known as a microscopist, asked for moral treatment in his handbook of 1865. Ludwig Traube did not believe in the psychogenic element in heart diseases in the beginning of his career, but was converted later (1867), and recommended, again according to the testimony of Leyden, psychotherapy in such cases. Ziemssen emphasized the psychogenic element in asthma and certain cases of heart disease. He was a partisan of the so-called neurasthenia theory, especially in gastrointestinal diseases. The neurasthenia theory spread primarily through the 1868 book of the New York clinician G. M. Beard. It covers largely the same field as the psychosomatics of today (see the book by E. Fischer-Homberger on hypochrondia).

Beneke and Carpenter were protagonists of a psychosomatic therapy and are quoted in this sense by J. Petersen. Ernst von Leyden observed psychogenic elements in diseases of the heart and stomach and in asthma, and recommended psychotherapy. Psychotherapy was also prescribed by the neurologist Erb, who is generally supposed to have been a supermechanist. F. A. Hoffmann accused anxiety of being a very important disease-producing element and asked for psychotherapy. Martius used hypnosis as well as suggestion. Ottomar Rosenbach discussed psychogenesis extensively and used psychotherapy just as much. It was of particular importance for the evolution in Germany that Strümpell, who for forty years influenced German clinicians very strongly through his textbook, published for the first time in 1883, was very open to psychosomatic ideas.

In certain diseases like heart disease, migraine, or thyrotoxicosis, Strümpell saw psychosomatic elements early. In others like asthma or peptic ulcer, he was converted to such a point of view only later through experience. In 1890, for example, he does not yet mention the psychogenic element in peptic ulcer, but he discusses it in 1917. Of other prominent, psychosomatically minded clinicians of that generation we would like to mention at least Stadelmann, Bruns, and especially Buttersack.

The psychosomatic element is quite obvious in gastroenterology, which developed between 1867 (gastric therapy with the stomach tube by Kussmaul) and 1886 (when Ismar Boas became the first practicing gastroenterologist in Berlin). The textbook of Ewald (1879), who, together with Leube (the latter still a partisan of the

notorious stomach brush of the seventeenth century!), laid the
foundations for gastroenterology, as well as the basic textbook of
Ismar Boas (1890) devote no less than one quarter of their space
to the so-called digestive neuroses. Numerous monographs of nervous diseases of the gastrointestinal tract were published during the
second half of the nineteenth century, such as those of Barras de
Fribourg, Beau, Trousseau, Budd, Spiller, O. Rosenthal, Oser. Very
successful was a small book by the Schaffhausen physician Alexander Peyer of 1890 on the connection between gastric disease and
male nervous diseases of the genital organs. Psychological treatment
was recommended even in books on pharmacology, e.g., those of
G. A. Richter (1826), Kraus (1862), D. Schroff (1862), and Oesterlen (1861).

Psychosomatic insight and therapeutics during the nineteenth century could be just as well demonstrated in British publications like
those by Sir Benjamin Brodie, Sir Astley Cooper, Langston Parker,
W. Stokes, J. H. Bennett, and M. MacKenzie.

The fairy tale, that clinicians lost psychosomatics during the nineteenth century all of a sudden, developed probably because psychosomatics, together with psychotherapy and the history of psychosomatics, is today no longer in the hands of internists but in the
hands of psychiatrists. These are in general even less familiar with
the history of internal medicine than with the history of their own
discipline.

It is undeniable that under the influence of so many new objective
discoveries and in a period of a firmer general attitude toward life,
psychosomatics was not so much in the limelight as today. Today
we are faced often with a hyperpsychosomatism, which is popular
because it provides easy and spectacular answers without great efforts. There was not as much noise around psychosomatics, but
psychosomatics was never lost. Unfortunately one thing has remained characteristic for this trend, i.e., its tendency to remain sta-
tionary and not to transgress certain elementary insights. Strümpell
said in 1922, rightly, that in this field often old wine filled new
and not always good bags.

Psychotherapy, as it developed after the end of the nineteenth
century, is a very interesting and to a large extent useful acquisition.
Within fifty years medicine changed from so-called psychophobia

(Eugen Bleuler) to so-called iatropsychology (Jerome Schneck). Schneck calls iatropsychology the trend, which tried now to answer all questions psychologically, in the fashion of the iatrophysicists or iatrochemists of the past, who, on the basis of insufficient scientific foundations, tried to explain everything either physically or chemically, and to treat it correspondingly. It is well known that modern psychotherapy derives from the methods of the Viennese physician Mesmer, who, in the 1770s, started treating with "animal magnetism." This magnetism of the treating physician was called "animal" in order to differentiate it from the treatment with the iron magnet. The German Romantics were enthusiastic partisans of Mesmerism, as was Hufeland. In the beginning of the nineteenth century several French Mesmerians, and especially the British surgeon James Braid, realized that this method actually did not mobilize physical, "magnetic" energies, but psychic ones. Braid therefore called the method hypnosis. Many practitioners used it, but it became more respectable only when, during the 1870s, two leading French clinicians, Jean Martin Charcot in Paris and Hippolyte Marie Bernheim in Nancy, adopted it. Then hypnosis became for a while a therapeutic fashion, only to be replaced by the "rational waking psychotherapy" of Paul Dubois and O. Rosenbach. The period around 1900 was in general a very active one in the field of psychotherapy and was rich in trends and methods.

Two men transgressed the pure hypnosis therapy and created the so-called cathartic therapy. One of them was Charcot's disciple Pierre Janet, who published in 1889 cases wherein he had succeeded in recalling during hypnosis forgotten traumatic memories and thus eliminated symptoms produced by these traumatic experiences. The Viennese internist and physiologist Joseph Breuer had had that experience as early as 1880. He published it only in 1893 together with his younger friend, the Viennese neurologist Sigmund Freud, who meanwhile had learned hypnosis with Charcot and Bernheim, and had become the translator of the works of both men. How Sigmund Freud transformed the cathartic method, around the turn of the century, into his psychoanalysis seems so well known that it is superfluous to give more details here. It is equally well known that from Freud's doctrine a number of similar doctrines branched off, which, taken altogether, are modern psychotherapy. Modern psychotherapy has been very useful, but it has also, in some quarters, become a mere fashion. In some Western centers today one is analyzed as one was clystered in the time of Molière. Some branches of modern psychotherapy have also taken an open stand against "inadequate science"; some function as new religions. Martini speaks rightly of the low-grade argumentation in Freud and his disciples. It is perhaps no accident that these doctrines are often popular today with people who exhibit in politics a similar quality of argumentation.

A special form of psychotherapy is musical therapy. Some kind of music (singing, drums, flutes, etc.) is an element of almost all magic rituals. In Greece musical therapy was secularized. Laymen as well as physicians practiced it. It did not entirely disappear in the Middle Ages. Baglivi and Kircher have transmitted to us the musical treatment of so-called tarantism in Apulia during the seventeenth century. During the eighteenth century a whole literature sprang up, which examined the therapeutic effect of music. These tendencies reappeared again and again in the nineteenth century.

XIII

Twentieth Century:
Chemotherapy, Antibiotics,
Hormones, Vitamins,
Psychopharmacology, Iatrogenic
Diseases

THE SERUM therapy of Behring had been a great success. This medicament had been a natural product; he had interpreted it in terms of a neohumoral pathology, and believed that it was impossible to duplicate this success in a purely chemical way. This was not the opinion of his collaborator, the Silesian Paul Ehrlich (1854–1915). In painstakingly detailed work, which lasted for decades, he accomplished this chemical deed. It seems justifiable to call Ehrlich a genius. Ehrlich was one of the last great men in medicine. Since Ehrlich we rather deal with middle-sized men. This undoubtedly is a consequence of the structural changes in science and society. Ehrlich was not only a great man, he was an extremely attractive character. As a Jew he could never be a full professor in the Germany of the Kaiser. He became in 1896 the director of an official institute for serum research in Steglitz and in 1899 director of an institute for experimental therapy in Frankfurt. This institute was enlarged tremendously in 1906 through a generous donation by the widow of George Speyer.

Ehrlich became famous primarily through his dye techniques in the fields of bacteriology and hematology, and furthermore through his research in immunity with toxic substances, which brought him the Nobel Prize in 1908. He is still remembered in the field of experimental cancer research. But his main claim to fame is probably his creation of chemotherapy.

All research endeavors of Ehrlich have come out of one single root. Even as a child he did experiments with dyeing flowers and animals in vivo. Whether he worked with Waldeyer in Strasbourg or in Leipzig with his cousin Weigert to take his doctorate, he always was primarily concerned with dyeing. Dyeing was so important to him because dyeing made visible a very basic problem—i.e., the problem of affinity between certain tissues and cells and certain chemicals. It is obvious that Ehrlich was very strongly influenced here through the cellular theory of Virchow, which he used consciously. Thus eventually a kind of cellular therapy came into being.

Ehrlich's ideas on immunity, as expounded in his Nobel lecture of 1908, were also the guideposts for his research in chemotherapy. In his opinion the molecules of toxin have "haptophores," side chains, which get anchored in the "chemoreceptors" of the cells of the body, another type of side chain. Antibodies are chemoreceptors which have been formed superabundantly. They fix the toxic haptophores and thus make them inactive. In analogy to these theories Ehrlich then tried to synthesize drug molecules, which contained haptophores which would attach themselves to the chemoreceptors of pathogenic microorganisms. In other words, Ehrlich tried to create artificial antitoxins or, to say it in his often poetic language, magic bullets. He tried to find preparations that were parasitotropic and not organotropic, i.e., that damage the parasite before they damage the patient. Ehrlich called this method "learn to aim through chemical variation," a method that is now used generally.

He began his chemotherapeutic experiments in 1904. In the beginning he used methylene blue against the plasmodia of malaria. Then, following Koch, he turned to fighting trypanosomes. He succeeded in 1904, together with Shiga, in discovering that trypan red was an effective medicament against tropical trypanosomes. The practical importance of this discovery for Germany was of a minor nature.

A much more urgent problem was the spirochetes, especially the causative organism of syphilis. Koch had used against syphilis an arsenical, the atoxyle of Béchamp, which was far too toxic to be successful. Arsenic had been, up to the seventeenth century, an antisyphilitic medicament. Ehrlich took up these old experiments of Koch's and succeeded, after years of experimenting with different arsenicals, in 1910 to find (together with the Japanese Hata) an arsenical called salvarsan or arsphenamine, which was an effective antisyphilitic. In the beginning Ehrlich and Hata called the preparation only Number 606, because it was the 606th chemical in these series of experiments. The toxicity of arsphenamine was within the limits of the tolerable. A later modification of arsphenamine, 912 or neoarsphenamine, was less toxic.

The echo produced by Ehrlich's discovery was tremendous, the hopes awakened limitless. Arsphenamine was not just an important and effective medicament against a very widespread and dangerous disease, it was the first in a long series of chemotherapeutics that were to follow it. This was a true specific. It attacked not only symptoms, it attacked the cause. It was not an accident, as quinine had been, but the result of systematic research started with a well-defined goal. The epoch of healing herbs was now definitely closed.

In the beginning all was not admiration for Ehrlich. Some of his colleagues formulated very strong doubts concerning his discovery. In addition mischievous anti-Semitic fools accused him of poisoning noble Aryan syphilitics out of low Jewish greediness. But they are all forgotten and Ehrlich's thought still influences pharmacological research very strongly.

In one respect Ehrlich's hopes and expectations were not fulfilled. He had hoped that he would be able to find a medicament that would at once destroy all microorganisms in the body of the patient (so-called therapia magna sterilisans). Ehrlich foresaw clearly the possibility of the evolution of drug-resistant organisms in a less radical form of treatment. Arsphenamine was not such a radically effective drug. It was therefore mostly combined with mercury or later bismuth. Three decades after its discovery it was replaced by penicillin, which is a far more effective and far less toxic substance.

Progress in the field of chemotherapy was not as rapid as had been hoped. During the two and a half decades after Ehrlich's great discovery no new successes could be registered except a few antimalarials, like atabrine and plasmochine, derived from dyes. Still no drugs against bacterial infections had been found. These became available in 1935 through the sulfanilamides. The sulfanilamides had long been known as dyes and were now introduced into therapeutics by Domagk. With the work of Domagk a new era of hopes, discoveries and successes starts in therapeutics. It was now possible to fight streptococci, the causative organisms of sepsis and puerperal fever, the staphylococci, the meningococci, the gonococci, and the pneumococci. In working with the sulfanilamides it became obvious that they very often did not kill the bacteria, as Ehrlich had wanted, but brought about only the so-called bacteriostasis; i.e., the bacteria were paralyzed and could then be destroyed by antibodies, leukocytes, etc.

The success of the sulfanilamides encouraged certain research men to go back to other bactericidal substances, which had not been followed up in that general atmosphere of disappointment which had so long hovered over chemotherapy. The bactericidal effect of molds, for example, had been known since the time of Pasteur. Attempts to prepare drugs from molds had been made repeatedly at the end of the nineteenth century. We mention only the experiments of Emmerich and Löw with pyocyanase in 1899 and of Gosio with penicillium in 1896. In 1929 Alexander Fleming had again demonstrated the bactericidal effect of the mold penicillium and had isolated from it penicillin.

In view of the menace of World War II, Florey and Chain in 1939 quickened their work with penicillin and brought it to a successful conclusion. Since then other antibiotics, e.g., streptomycin, aureomycin, chloromycetin, have been isolated from such fungi. With their help not only the infections previously mentioned but also plague, tuberculosis, and even rickettsial diseases can be therapeutically influenced. Against most of the viral diseases these preparations seem ineffective. But the general progress is tremendous.

Where there is much light, there is also much shadow. We have been forced by experience to admit that the antibiotics are not at all always as harmless as it was originally assumed. The worst is that antibiotic-resistant strains, especially penicillin-resistant staphylococci, have developed, which make therapeutics sometimes quite difficult and which have brought about a renaissance of the horrible "hospitalism" of a hundred years ago. Partly responsible for this situation is the entirely uncritical use of antibiotics, which was customary for a while and has still not yet died out. Dickinson W. Richards (Nobel Prize, 1956) has rightly stated that antibiotics have often brought about a certain sloppiness in practice, as many physicians no longer diagnose before giving antibiotics nor follow up the patient once they have given antibiotics. A form of therapy has developed which Wuhrmann has justifiably called "hurrah"-therapy. One could also call this automatic routine—which, without any thought, reacts to certain symptoms simply by giving antibiotics, or cortisone, or tranquilizers—"reflex"-therapy. Another negative aspect of the success of the antibiotics is that all those microorganisms that they do not affect can grow all the better, and infections with those organisms, which were once rare or unknown, have now become very widespread.

In spite of all, progress is enormous. A 1935 book by a Zurich practitioner, Dr. O. Fiertz, *What Is Still Useful after 40 Years?* shows us the customary armamentarium of a practitioner of the first quarter of the century. Fiertz still very often gave calomel. Salol was for him, as for others, a panacea. He frequently gave camphor and tried cupping in pleurisy. He liked Nägeli's manipulations in neurotics and salt-free diet. He recommended arsacetine and almateine, but opposed the much-used creosote.

In order to visualize the whole evolution of therapeutics since 1921, we list here those 20 medicaments that Huchard and Fiessinger, in their excellent book, *Therapeutics with 20 Medicaments,* discussed in the fifth edition of 1921: aspirin, quinine, mercury, potassium iodide, digitalis, iron, sera and vaccines, collargol, hormones, theobromine, bismuth, sodium bicarbonate, arsenic, opium, belladonna, potassium bromide, cathartics, nitrates, ergot, and antipyrine.

Of hormones, actually only thyroid gland preparations were known at this moment. The enormous progress in hormone research during the twentieth century just began at this moment thanks to collaboration with the biochemists. Today pharmacology and biochemistry have become inseparable. The great hormone discovery of 1921—the isolation of insulin by F. G. Banting and his collaborators —made so far incurable diabetes an object of therapeutics. In the beginning of the 1930s the chemical nature of the male and female sexual hormones was elucidated by Butenandt and others. Sexual hormones have since been often used therapeutically. Huggins in 1966 received the Nobel Prize for treating cancer of the prostate with female sexual hormones. Female sexual hormones were unfortunately given quite uncritically in general gynecological difficulties and produced fatal tumors. Since the middle of the 1930s Reichstein, Kendall, and others worked with adrenal hormones, and adrenal hormones have now found an important place in therapeutics. They passed through a period of overenthusiastic misuse as so many other drugs had before. Work with the hormones of the hypophysis also proved very successful.

The twentieth century has been the century of vitamin research. Empirically scurvy had been treated for a long time with citrus fruits or beriberi, since Takaki (1882), with a mixed diet. But insight into the nature of vitamins developed only out of the experimental work of Eijkman (1897), F. G. Hopkins (1906), and C. Funk (1912). Vitamins A, B, and D were now discovered by MacCollum, Steenbock, Osborn, Mendel, Windaus, and others in the years following 1913. Of great practical importance were the experiments of J. Goldberger with pellagra after 1914. No empirical pellagra treatment had been known before. Of far greater practical importance for our latitudes was the fact that on the basis of the knowledge of avitaminosis, now rickets could be prevented and treated. The same holds good for the treatment of beriberi in the Far East, which is based above all on the work of R. R. Williams in the Philippines. We do not want to hide here the fact that the commercial exploitation of the discovery of vitamins degenerated into a vigorous attack on the pocketbooks of credulous hypochondriacs. Some have therefore called vitamins the most expensive placebos. The discovery of George Richard Minot in 1926 that raw liver is an effective drug in pernicious anemia, which, up to that time, had been always fatal, is also basically a vitamin discovery. Today pernicious anemia is treated directly with vitamin B_{12}.

Reasons of space make it impossible to even only mention here all the new medicaments of the last decades. Anyhow many of them are not yet proper objects of history. But we would like to mention at least the antithyroids, which were introduced in the 1930s, and the sulfones and PAS, used against tuberculosis. In view of the frequency of coronary infarction the development of anticoagulants like heparin (Jarpes), dicumarol (K. P. Link), etc., was of great practical importance. Antihistamines, used against allergies, were developed by Bovet (1937) and Halpern (1942). The team of Bovet-Nitti had unveiled before, with Tréfouel, the sulfa riddle. Bovet was given the Nobel Prize in 1957 for his work on the blocking of muscle stimulants. The discovery of the spirolactones (antialdosterones) has given us new, effective, nonmercurial diuretics. The twentieth century has brought us also a series of successful vaccinations: BCG in 1921, antidiphtheria and antitetanus vaccination (Ramon, 1923), vaccinations against yellow fever, typhus, whooping cough in the 1940s, the polio vaccinations by Salk and Sabin in the 1950s. Worthy of mention also is the distribution of iodized salt in goiter regions and the fluoridation of the drinking water as a prophylactic against caries. We must abstain here from giving details of the development of traditional pharmacological problems like the preparation of the glycosides of digitalis by Cloetta (1920), Windaus (1928), and Stoll (1930). In general not only the old traditional plant drugs but also the old mineral drugs have disappeared.

We have entered the era of macromolecules. When great masses of people are pensioned off, unavoidably once in a while individuals who are still very vigorous are retired. That holds true for pharmaka too.

The first effective somatic treatment of a mental disease was the malaria treatment of general paresis by J. von Wagner-Jauregg in 1917. Thereafter for many years a great number not only of mental diseases but also of other diseases were treated with fever—unfortunately with little success. This pyretic wave of nonspecific stimuli, which dominated the 1920s and 1930s, is not a glorious leaf in the history of therapeutics. We witnessed this reedition of Brownism only forty years ago. Proteins were used, for example, in infectious diseases like gonorrhea, influenza, pneumonia, dysentery, typhoid fever, scarlet fever, sepsis, puerperal fever, anthrax, meningitis. The same substances were used against arthritis, obesity, allergies, peptic ulcer, as well as neurosyphilis, neuralgia, neuritis, and multiple sclerosis. The latter was also fought with collargol, which at that time functioned as a panacea.

Other somatic methods of treating mental disease were the different shock treatments of Sakel (1933), Meduna (1935), and Cerletti and Bini (1938). In 1936 Moniz and Lima introduced prefrontal lobotomy. Fortunately since the beginning of the 1950s the emphasis in somatic psychiatric treatment has been on pharmacological-chemical methods. The first preparations of this group were descendants of the classic Hindu drug, rauwolfia, or of chloropromazine, an antihistamine. Meanwhile a new discipline, psychopharmacology, has developed. So far no causal treatment has been possible in this field, but everybody who has known the old agitated wards of psychiatric clinics or asylums is profoundly impressed by the change these drugs have brought about. The abuse of them by many physicians and laymen is regrettable. New drugs have also been found for a more effective treatment of parkinsonism and epilepsy.

The essential difference between past and present is not in the total quantity of the medicaments available. There have always been numerous medicaments, and, of course, industry multiplies their number continuously. In the United States, for example, annually 300 to 400 new medicaments are brought to the market. What is different today is the quantity of effective products. These entitle us actually to state that since the 1930s an era of successful prevention has been replaced by an era of successful therapeutics. The disturbing aspect of this era is the very great number of medicaments, which in the course of one disease are given to one patient, the new polypharmacy.

Drugs are more reliable because, since 1945, the placebo experiments and double blind tests have been used systematically. Physiological-experimental methods, together with clinical control and statistics, had at the end of the nineteenth century produced such solid acquisitions as hormones, antisera, and chemotherapy. Nevertheless the need for new methods of objective appraisal of therapeutic results had not yet been satisfied. Pinel had emphasized the psychological difficulties that lay in the way of an objective assessment of therapeutic results. He had written about those who confound the illusions of their imagination with reality, and who ignore the secret influence of their prejudices. To the extent that the development of science reduced the objective difficulties of therapeutic progress, these subjective impediments became particularly obvious. The placebo experiment was introduced into research in order to avoid these pitfalls. It had been given attention as early as 1891 by O. Rosenbach, who was as strange a thinker as he was ingenious. Rosenbach, by the way, also predicted molecular pathology. The placebo effect had, of course, been known for a long time in therapeutics and had been used consciously by clinicians like Lind, Andral, or Bernheim. The most surprising result of placebo research is perhaps that placebos do not only cure but also produce "toxic" side effects.

In spite of all progress in research it must be stated that the relations between structure and effect still are by no means clear. It is equally obvious that medicaments have become more dangerous to the extent that they have become more effective. It is assumed today that from 5 to 20 percent of hospital inmates suffer from iatrogenic disease. In view of the great number of medicaments given to one individual, it is often very difficult to find out which one produced the damage. On the other hand, illusions concerning the quantity of iatrogenic diseases in the past are unwarranted. It is true, most of the ancient medicaments were not very effective, but iatrogenic anemia and iatrogenic mercury poisoning were extremely widespread.

The advances of surgery are, due to the mass media, so well known and so numerous that we will not discuss them here. We will, on the other hand, at least mention a new field of therapeutics that came into being at the beginning of the century. Since 1896 x-rays and since 1905 the radiation of radium have been used therapeutically, especially against cancerous diseases. In the past two decades radioactive isotopes have been used more and more in therapeutics. Milder forms of radiation therapy in the first half of the twentieth century were ultraviolet irradiation and diathermy.

Those who, as laymen or physicians, have witnessed the past fifty years, have seen the appearance and disappearance of numerous therapeutic fashions, which were no longer spontaneous, but were produced by sales propaganda and unscrupulous journalism. Many of the medicaments mentioned previously were for a while rather dangerous fashionable drugs and panaceas. Certain pathological theories produced surgical fashions like Bier's venous congestion, the surgical fight against "focal infections" or discopathies, which are no longer used so frequently. Socialist Russia provided several therapeutic fashions, like the rejuvenation serum of Bogomolets and the pumping of the cerebrospinal fluid by Speransky. Yet dying Stalin was treated with leeches. For a while everything became a panacea: vitamins, steroids, antibiotics, antihistamines, psychopharmaceuticals, etc. What will be the next panacea? Or will we be favored with a reduction of the panacea tendency and the new polypharmacy? Will the computer be helpful in this direction?

Lasègue was undoubtedly right when writing a hundred years ago: "Not pathological discoveries, but general theories, basic doctrines, general trends of opinion, direct therapeutics." It seems nevertheless that with the progress of objectivation a certain change has occurred, and therapeutic discussions are more often concerned with technical details, not with general theories. One method of objectivation, the self-experiment of the physician, has by no means disappeared in this last phase of therapeutics. We can cite the curare self-experiments of S. M. Smith, the self-experiments with different vaccinations (Shaughnessy and others, the collaborators of J. Salk, etc.), Frischmuth's self-experiments with sulfanilamides, and those of A. Hofmann with LSD.

Additional Remarks On the History of Iatrogenic Disease

The problem of iatrogenic disease seems so important that we would like to return to it once more. We know not only of detrimental effects of indifferent or harmful medicaments, which we have reported repeatedly. There do unfortunately exist also the pathogenic consequences and side effects of medicaments that are very valuable.

In the course of the past decade at least half a dozen books and innumerable articles have appeared dealing with these "iatrogenic diseases." The catastrophic effects of thalidomide have brought to the knowledge of a larger public what physicians have known for a long time, i.e., that effective medicaments can have very dangerous side effects. Iatrogenic diseases of the skin, the blood (especially since W. Schultz described agranulocytosis in 1922), the liver, the kidney, the gastrointestinal tract, the eye and the ear, the endocrine glands, the nervous system including the soul, and the so-called electrolyte balance have been described. Iatrogenic collagen diseases, infections, and malignant tumors are known. Old medicaments, like mercurials, digitalis, organic combinations of arsenic or gold, even oxygen still cause diseases. For decades damage produced by irradiation, by salicylates, and by transfusions has been observed. But the larger part of new iatrogenic diseases has been observed in connection with the use of sulfanilamides and antibiotics, which otherwise have been so useful. The corticosteroids are known to produce numerous pathological side effects. Psychopharmaceuticals are not as harmless as was assumed originally. Chloropromazine, for example, has in some cases been responsible for such various diseases as parkinsonism, aplastic anemia, icterus, damage of the retina, and arrhythmias. Antihypertonics, especially the ganglion-blocking ones, can be pathogenic. The same holds true for anticoagulants, anticonvulsants, antirheumatics, and contrast substances. Cytostatics are a high risk. These have been the main results of the study of iatrogenic disease during the past years.

Iatrogenic diseases themselves are old, probably as old as therapeutics, and have been recognized for a long time. New is probably their greater frequency in connection with the discovery of more effective medicaments. New is furthermore the interest in the subject. New is eventually the term, which reflects the facts mentioned above, and the increasingly scientific character of our medicine.

In former chapters it has become obvious that diseases that were objectively iatrogenic have been known in the past. In view of the importance of the problem, it seems necessary to survey briefly the question in adding new details.

Louis Lewin reports in his *History of Poisons* famous cases of iatrogenic disease and death, such as the death of one of the friends of emperor Nero through cantharides, that of Otto II from aloe, that of Gregorius from colchicine, of Avicenna through a combination of pepper clysters and opium. Henry I and Amalrich too were killed by cantharides, while the death of Voltaire was attributed to opium. It is obvious that the centuries old use and misuse not only of cathartics and emetics but especially of bloodletting must have had again and again fatal consequences. Two iatrogenic infections that devastated hospitals up to the middle of the nineteenth century were typhus, especially in the wards for internal diseases, and septicemia in surgery and obstetrics. They induced Leibniz to call the hospitals of his time *seminaria mortis*.

In view of these facts physicians have, from Hippocrates through the Alexandrians and Asklepiades to Galen, been critical of certain methods of treatment. The old Hindus knew the harmful consequences of too much bleeding, cathartics, and emetics. Such critical remarks are also known from the Middle Ages, the Arabic as well as the Western Middle Ages. Pietro d'Argellato pointed toward the detrimental effects of iodine-containing goiter medicaments. In view of the underdeveloped state of medicine in these epochs, it is of course not always clear whether actually iatrogenic disease was observed, or whether wrong diagnoses were made.

Discussions of detrimental side effects of drugs become more and more numerous in modern times. For the sixteenth century we have quoted the polemics of Paracelsus against contemporary therapeutics, especially with mercury. We have mentioned the antimercurialism, i.e., the protest against the abuse of mercury in the treatment of syphilis, beginning with Fernelius in the sixteenth century. The same tendency can be observed during the next century. The most radical critic of disease-producing therapeutics in the seventeenth century was van Helmont. But even Sydenham, who was certainly no niggard in the use of mercury, knew that hysteria and dropsy can appear after too much bloodletting and purging. Peruvian bark was attacked very violently (and partly without foundation) by Gideon Harvey and others. It is characteristic for the spirit of the century that Ettmüller calls his treatise of 1661 on so-called precipitants, to which the bark belonged, not a treatise on the use of precipitants, but on the use and misuse of precipitants.

At the beginning of the eighteenth century the famous Boerhaave believed that rabies might be caused by too much bleeding and purging, while he explained cases of scurvy through abuse of the bark. Complaints concerning the bad effect of therapeutically used phosphorus and arsenic became so numerous in the early eighteenth century that these medicaments were given only rarely. Gaub, the successor of Boerhaave, has, in his book on pathology, a whole chapter on "the unreasonable use of medicaments."

In the beginning of the eighteenth century the first monographs on iatrogenic diseases appear. In 1726 the Halle clinician G. E. Stahl published his *Examination of Badly Cured and Spoiled Diseases*. Stahl here condenms cathartics, emetics, sudorifics, and especially opium, the use of which, according to him, produces hectic fevers, dropsy, cachexia, colics, and gout. Mercury and several medicaments used against epilepsy he thinks to be very harmful. Treatment with gold is swindle to him, and the panacea Peruvian bark extremely dangerous. He also feels that spas are misused as well as astringents and iron medication.

Frederic Hoffmann, Stahl's colleague and competitor in Halle, defends the same opinions. His opuscula of 1736 contain three pamphlets dealing with the subject. In the first, "Unwise Medication as a Cause of Many Diseases and Death," Hoffmann examines the wrong use of venesection, emetics, drastics, sudorifics, opium, and mercurials. Like Stahl he condemns astringents because they stop hemorrhages, especially from the hemorrhoids which they both thought to be so very wholesome. He also refused the bark. He believed that physicians use wrong medicaments on account of a too violent temperament. In his second pamphlet, "On the Misuse and the Damage Arising from the Application of the Mild Medicaments," he goes even farther, often too far. Water, wine, sweets, milk, hot infusions, cold drinks might do harm. The same holds for the suppression of nosebleed and the suppression of pain in rheumatism. Tea, coffee, and chocolate might be just as harmful as heavy meals in fever, meat in head traumatism, sweets in stomach disease (the latter observation had been made before him). Further damage could be produced through the use of milk, oils, fats, footbaths and other baths, neutral salts, acids, liquor, and moschus. In a third pamphlet he discusses the "Ordinary Errors in the Application of Local Remedies in Practice."

During the eighteenth century Halle seems to have been a center for studying iatrogenic diseases. A whole series of doctoral dissertations were published there dealing with the subject, such as that of G. E. Weiss of 1728, "Doctors as the Cause of Disease," which, on the basis of case histories, analyzes the detrimental effects of bleeding and antimony. Other dissertations covering this field were submitted by Zweifel in 1701, Curtius in 1714, Zeys in 1722, Langguth in 1739, Kühne in 1763, and Schlenther in 1777. J. Lenhardt, who published in Leipzig in 1788 his *Medicaments without Mask,* had studied in Halle. Prominent members of the Halle faculty were J. Ch W. Juncker and J. Ch. Reil, who both in their general works pay much attention to the iatrogenic damage or, as it was called in the past, side effects of therapeutics (1791 and 1799). August Friedrich Hecker, who did the same in his general pathology of 1791, was another former Halle student.

This Halle tradition continued even into the next century with Curt Sprengel who, in his handbook of pathology (Leipzig 1802), extensively described the "abuse of medicaments as a cause of diseases." Reminiscences of Stahl are obvious. In addition Sprengel discusses new drugs, like cherry laurel, nightshade, hyoscyamus, hemlock, and digitalis. The study of iatrogenic diseases was, of course, not limited to Halle. In 1775 there appeared for instance in London a book by Thomas Withers of Edinburgh, *Observations on the Misuse of Medicaments.* Withers criticized here the abuse of bleeding, emetics, purging, sudorifics, so-called stimulants, mercury, opium, tea, coffee, and bark. Surprisingly enough he was rather uncritical in the use of cantharides.

The nineteenth century too studied iatrogenic diseases. In the 1820s therapeutic intoxications with bromine and iodine were described. Other new drugs were examined in this direction, or the toxic effects of older medicaments were analyzed. The famous German clinician Kussmaul dealt repeatedly with such problems, as in the case of mercury or of bloodletting. But for a longer period no general books on this subject appeared. In addition the respective chapters disappeared from the general works on pathology. Only at the end of the century did the unforgettable Louis Lewin publish his *Side Effects of Medicaments* (Berlin, 1881). The literature on iatrogenic diseases here makes a new start. Lewin uses the then customary and long-prevailing name of "side effects." The name sounds milder than toxic. I do not know why general works on iatrogenic diseases disappeared for a certain period and whether this gap can be connected with the then arising therapeutic nihilism. Even therapeutic nihilism can, as Hans Fischer remarks, become, paradoxically enough, the cause of iatrogenic disease. In any case Lewin's book coincides with a strong activation in medication.

Lewin tries first a general theory of side effects, their connection with the individual, with time and place, and with the constitution of the medicament. He states that drugs that are effective unavoidably have side effects, but that side effects can be limited through chemical change of the drug. He then examines the drugs in detail, still using the old-fashioned subdivision into tonics, astringents, alterants, narcotics, etc. His list of side effects is, of course, simultaneously a list of the then most frequently used medicaments and interesting also from this point of view. Particularly strong side effects are reported (he has surveyed the whole literature) with quinine and salicylates. They play a lesser role in strychnine and turpentine, while copaiba balm and bismuth show more undesirable consequences. Argyrism is very widespread as a sequel of the use of silver preparations in epilepsy and locomotor ataxia. Lead, zinc oxide, and barium chloride (then a specific against scrofula) produce only moderate intoxications. The same holds good for ergot, used then primarily against fibromyoma.

Carbolism was, of course, very widespread during these years. Carbolic acid was used not only as a disinfectant but also in internal medicine. Senator, for example, injected carbolic acid into articulations in polyarthritis. Many therapeutic intoxications with mercury, arsenic, iodine, bromine (especially the bromism of epileptics) were reported. Opium and belladonna produced numerous side effects. Fewer side effects were observed with camphor, aconite, veratrine, colchicine, and digitalis. Frequent sources of disagreeable phenomena were chloral hydrate, chloroform, and ether. Tartar emetic, still applied as an ointment on the head of mentally diseased people, might have toxic effects on the heart. In the case of santonin, pilocarpine, cantharides, chrysarobine, one should not be surprised by negative side effects. It will not have escaped the attention of the reader that a high percentage of these substances have disappeared from practical use during the past ninety years.

The next book on the side effects of modern drugs was produced by Otto Seifert and appeared in Würzburg in 1915, a supplement in 1922. Subdivisions are here far more modern: antipyretics, anesthetics, heart drugs, gastrointestinal drugs, etc. We can report here only some data from this work. As with Lewin, damage done by antipyretics plays a great role. While in 1881 the salicylates were mostly responsible, now antifebrine, antipyrine, phenacetin, and pyramidon are the culprits. Among anesthetics ethyl bromine (liver damage), cocaine, chloroform, sulfonal, and veronal seem the most dangerous. Among heart drugs this role is played by digitalis, among gastrointestinal drugs oleum chenopodii, among urinary drugs salol. Emetine constipates only. The author avoids a discussion of salvarsan (arsphenamine). In skin diseases he cautions against cacodyle (also applied in tuberculosis) and atoxyle. He furthermore deals extensively with iodine preparations, with collargol and lysol. In the second volume, appearing after the influenza epidemic of 1918, he reports the frequent catastrophic damage done by optochine.

In 1922 Strümpell, the dean of German clinicians, discussed our subject in the *Deutsche Medizinische Wochenschrift.* Strümpell feels that after the end of therapeutic nihilism a new tide of therapeutic hyperactivity has arisen. Strümpell attacks his polypragmasy and points toward sublimate, carbolic acid, iodoform, arsphenamine, optochine, and sulfonal as drugs that are particularly apt to produce detrimental side effects. Hypochondria can also be, with him, a kind of iatrogenic disease, as certain physicians are producing it on a large scale.

It is impossible to discuss in detail here all the reports on the side effects of tuberculin, insulin, mesothorium, etc. A third wave of general occupation with iatrogenic diseases began in the 1950s, as mentioned at the beginning of this chapter. Recently several authors have underlined the fact that preventive measures offer in general less danger of iatrogenic disease than therapeutic activities. Peter Waser is right in saying: "Pharmacotherapy is always a calculated risk, just like an operation."

XIV

Final Discussion

LOOKING BACK at the long history of therapeutics we realize that it by no means followed a straight line. Periods of great activity have been followed by periods of lesser activity. Often therapeutics stagnated. Often it turned in a circle. Occasionally the spirit of invention was quite active. What is altogether striking is the relative permanence, not to say the monotony, of therapeutic techniques, while at the same time pathological theories appeared and disappeared continuously.

Certain negative traits, which seem to be deeply rooted in human psychology, have been in evidence at all times. First is a well-meant but uncritical activism which at best has positive psychological effects. No less fatal is an arrogant activism as we have seen, for example, with the Galenists. This attitude is closely connected with an uncritical conservatism. The old as such is regarded as a value, and through the centuries traditions which often have been directly harmful are handed down thoughtlessly. Certain therapeutic activities appear to the outsider as if they were meant to be punishments.

The counterpart of the just-mentioned adoration of the old, or paleophilia, which has now become rarer, is neophilia, the uncritical acceptance of everything new. "What is new, is good." Corvisart made fun of this attitude with his famous saying: "This remedy is new. Take it rapidly as long as it is still curative." In this attitude lies also one of the roots of present polypharmacy. In hunting hastily the new, one loses all too easily something old that was good. Even the new that is good is often paid for dearly with sacrifices as we have seen in the history of digitalis, iodine, quinine, and the mineral-chemical drugs.

It is amazing to see to what extent fashion has played a role in therapeutics. As early as 1713 the French playwright Destouches spoke of medical fashions. Very different medical thinkers like G. Wedekind, A. F. Hecker, and G. L. Bayle recognized very clearly at the beginning of the nineteenth century the existence of medical fashions. The *Dictionnaire des Sciences Médicales* had a special chapter on them, and mentioned as the therapeutic fashions of 1819: electricity, magnetism, phosphorus, ether, sulfur baths, copaiba balm, steam baths, and moxa. It is, by the way, obvious that not only therapeutics but also diagnostics are influenced by fashion.

We have seen that even the reign of true scientific attitudes in other areas of medicine has not excluded the existence of such mistakes in therapeutics. Psychotherapeutics resembles somatic, non-surgical therapeutics in this respect. The lack of a critical attitude might even be more pronounced in this domain. It is in the nature of things that surgery has been often more solid in its attitudes. But a more detailed examination of the history of surgery shows that surgery too has suffered a great deal from the evils mentioned above. The "hurrah"-surgery can be encountered just as often as the "hurrah"-therapy.

It is understandable that, under these circumstances, for 2500 years again and again the slogan "back to Hippocrates" has been voiced. Hippocrates symbolizes a reserved, expectative, modest attitude confiding in nature. Science has given us during the past decades so many extremely effective and valuable substances that it would be not only reactionary but senseless and unscrupulous to return simply to expectative or nihilistic attitudes. The whole history of therapeutics seems nevertheless to suggest to therapists, pushed from all sides into unbridled activity, a certain sensible reserve as it is connected with the name of Hippocrates. Too often one has relied on the extraordinary toughness of the human organism. It is not completely irrelevant either that polypharmacy is very expensive.

With the help of pathology and physiological chemistry we have succeeded, during the past 150 years, in making therapeutics more objective and have gone beyond the limits of symptomatic treatment. Therapeutics is nevertheless still in a certain sense an "art," an "art of the possible," as Kartagener has called it. But this should be no reason to adopt "intensely artistic attitudes," attitudes where "all too often the cloven foot of the quack does not remain hidden."

Before ending this discussion I would like to look at the motives that induce therapists to apply this or that technique, to be expectative or active. Immediately the hypothesis imposes itself that therapeutics depends basically on the general scientific world view of the therapist, especially whether this view is vitalistic or mechanistic.

If we start by applying this hypothesis to Greek medicine, it seems to be confirmed. The basic idea of most Hippocratic writings is that in men a powerful force, the so-called physis, nature, is active which brings about the cure. The Hippocratic writings, like those of Aristotle, are vitalistic. If nature cures, the role of the physician is not that of the leader, but of the servant of nature, who helps to restore through a mild, expectative, mostly dietetic therapy the balance of humors.

If we go one step farther and examine physicians dominated by nonvitalistic ancient ideas, by the mechanistic theories of a Democritus or Epicurus, we discover indeed that, e.g., the first known solidist in medical history, the Alexandrian Erasistratus, was logically enough a very aggressive therapist. With him no physis brought about cure.

When, during the Renaissance, Hippocratism was revived by men like Baillou, Cesalpino, Valleriola, and J. Lange, expectative therapy again gained ground. Even of the English Hippocratist Thomas Sydenham it can be said that he was at least a less aggressive therapist than most of his contemporaries. The famous Leiden iatrochemist, Sylvius (De le Boë), was, on the other hand, logical in being a very active therapist, as he did not believe in the healing power of nature.

The tendency toward expectative treatment is very clear with the promoter of neovitalism during the eighteenth century, G. E. Stahl, and the vitalistic Hippocratists of Montpellier, like Bordeu and Pinel, whom he influenced.

Unfortunately, in spite of these beautiful confirmations of our hypothesis, we find at closer examination so many deviations that it has to be abandoned. General biological opinions might have formed therapy occasionally. As a rule they do not. If biological theories would automatically rule therapeutics, it would not be necessary to write a special history of therapeutics. It could be easily derived from the general history of medical theories. Our problem was examined in 1844 by a medical writer, P. Reinbold, who otherwise did not gain fame. In analyzing the activities of his contemporaries he concluded that vitalistic convictions by no means exclude therapeutic activism, and that an expectative attitude can be observed with physicians who do not recognize the healing power of nature as a principle.

The first great example of a mechanist and antivitalist, who as a practitioner was rather expectative and reasonable, is Asklepiades, whom we have described before. Galen, on the other hand, always emphatically designated himself as a Hippocratist and a vitalist. He gave enthusiastic descriptions of the healing power of nature. But as a practitioner he was an all too eager "servant of nature" and an incorrigible polypharmacist. Neuburger rightly defined Galenism as a combination of extensive drug treatment and theoretical recognition of nature as a healer.

Galen is only the acme of an evolution toward activating therapeutics which fills the whole post-Hippocratic period and which Asklepiades failed to stop. The Alexandrian empiricists gave more drugs but bled less. The methodists gave less drugs but more physical therapy. Celsus bled more and gave less medicaments. Galen and his followers bled, gave drugs, purged, and used physical therapy. It is therefore not surprising that prominent Galenists of the Renaissance like Botallo, Riolan, Guy Patin, and Mercurialis were particularly overactive therapists.

On the other hand, the great anti-Galenist of the Renaissance, Paracelsus, who abounded in lip service to the healing power of nature, was just as aggressive a therapist. The same holds true for his great disciple van Helmont. He was a vitalist, but, as a physician, he wanted to be "rector" and not "minister" of nature. He abandoned quite a number of activistic techniques, like bleeding, purging, fontanelles, etc., but used all the more antimony and sudorific drugs.

The seventeenth and eighteenth centuries exhibit not only the aggressive vitalists but also the expectative mechanists like Baglivi, Boerhaave, and Frederic Hoffmann. It is not surprising that at the end of the eighteenth century Hippocratists, like Tronchin and Pinel, favor expectation. But it must be admitted that the mechanist Corvisart and his disciples defend a very similar point of view. At the same time hyperactivity in its most repulsive forms is represented by vitalists like Brown, Rasori, Reil, Broussais, and Bouillaud.

What then are the actual motives that influence therapists? It is extremely difficult to gain clarity in this respect, as the arguments of therapists are very often products of self-deception or what the psychoanalysts call rationalization. Significant in this respect is that the same drugs and operations have been used for centuries with very different justifications. Temkin, in a study on the therapeutic tendencies in syphilis treatment before 1900 (*Bull. History Medicine 29:* 309–316, 1955), named four factors that influence therapeutics:

1. Empirical factors, i.e., knowledge of the disease and of the therapeutic and toxic effects of drugs. In this connection he mentions analogy, which has a tremendous influence in therapeutics.
2. General theories. A very impressive example in this respect is the salivation in mercury treatment, which is based on humoralism.
3. Economic and social motives.
4. Religious and moral motives.

It is in the nature of things that the first point of Temkin, empirical factors, rarely are derived from individual experience. "Experience" rules the therapeutics of the physician in the form of "tradition," i.e., a mixture that pretends to reflect the experience of the whole profession. My colleague, H. M. Koelbing, prefers to call this collective experience "esprit de corps," as the drugs and methods under discussion are very often not old, but brand new. He underlines the fact that, in order to be accepted by the practitioners, a recommendation of a drug by large hospitals or leading colleagues is decisive. The same drug, if recommended only by outsiders, is not accepted in general. Eugen Bleuler fifty years ago gave in his *Autistic-Undisciplined Thought* a critical analysis of subjective elements in our collective behavior, which unfortunately is far from being outdated. The same holds for his statement "the more one approaches therapeutics, the more scientific acumen is abandoned in favor of the use of a sometimes excellent, sometimes very mediocre common sense." Eventually the personal temperament of the therapist undoubtedly plays a role in his therapeutic decisions.

Dominant general theories may influence therapeutics, but they do not necessarily have this effect, as we have seen in the case of cellular theory. The same holds for dominant diseases, which do not necessarily exert a general influence on therapeutics.

The public is a partner in the therapeutic decisions of physicians who is as important as he is often forgotten. Certainly fashions, so characteristic for the history of therapeutics, are partly produced by the physicians themselves. But to a very large extent they generate under the pressure of the patients. Patients have a strange inclination toward "magic procedures," or they interpret scientific procedures as magic. It seems that the irrational is psychologically more satisfactory than the rational. History also shows patient and physician again and again as willing victims of propaganda.

Some have seen in therapeutics a direct expression of the lifestyle of the epoch. It is very difficult to prove this in detail. Motives in therapeutics are an extremely complex mixture, which reflects, on the one hand, developments in medicine and science, and on the other hand, external factors.

My picture of the therapeutics of our time has probably been too rosy. But it seems to me that for the therapeutic future we can be very hopeful, at least as far as single problems like the treatment of cancer are concerned. A general tendency toward specific therapy and molecular therapy seems predominant now. Many new problems of therapeutics will be partly problems of care (e.g., in geriatrics). Further objectivation will be necessary (e.g., in the field of psychotherapy). The computer will undoubtedly play a great role in the process of greater objectivation. A certain skepticism still seems necessary even to the modern therapist in view of the production of innumerable new drugs and their unrestrained praise through an often unscrupulous publicity and in view of the tendencies toward panaceas and polypharmacy.

Our history of therapeutics has often been rather critical. I hope it has always remained clear that this was done without any petty feelings of superiority in relation to our predecessors. On the contrary they still deserve our full gratitude.

Bibliography

ACKERKNECHT, E. H.: Natural diseases and rational treatment in primitive medicine. Bull. Hist. Med. 19: 467–497, 1946. — id.: Medical Practices. Handbook Southamerican Indian. 5: 621–643, Washington 1949. — id.: Aspects of the History of Therapeutics. Bull. Hist. Med. 36: 389–419, 1962. — id.: Panazeen in Documenta Geigy; Fundamente moderner Medizin, S. 8, 1964. — id.: Kurze Geschichte der Medizin. Durchgesehene Ausgabe, Stuttgart 1967. — id.: Medicine at the Paris Hospital 1794–1848. Baltimore 1967. — id.: Zellulartheorie und-therapie. Praxis 57: 126–127, 1968. — id.: Therapeutische Selbstversuche. Documenta Geigy, S. 5–6, 1969. — id.: Die therapeutische Erfahrung und ihre allmähliche Objektivierung. Gesnerus 26: 28–35, 1969.

BAUER, K. J.: Geschichte der Aderlässe. Munich 1870. — BERMAN, A.: The Heroic Approach in 19th Century Therapeutics. Bull. Am. Soc. Hosp. Pharm. Sept. 1954, 320–327. — BLEULER, E.: Das autistisch-undisziplinierte Denken in der Medizin und seine Ueberwindung. Berlin 1919. — BROCKBANK, W.: Ancient Therapeutic Arts. London 1954. — BRUPPACHER-CELLIER, M.: Rudolf Buchheim (1820–79). Zurich 1971. — BUESS, H.: Die historischen Grundlagen der intravenösen Injektion. Aarau 1946. — id.: Die Injektion. Ciba Zeitschrift No. 100, März 146. — BYNUM, W.: Chemical Structure and Pharmaceutic Effect. Bull. Hist. Med. 44: 518–38, 1970.

CABANÈS: Remèdes d'autrefois. Paris 1910. — COLWELL, A. A.: A History of Electrotherapy, London 1922.

DUBLER, C. E.: Die "Materia Medica" unter den Muslimen des Mittelalters. Sudhoffs Archiv 43: 329–350, 1959.

EARLES, M. P.: Experiments with Drugs and Poisons in the 17th and 18th Centuries. Ann. of Sc. 19: 245–254, 1963. — EBSTEIN, E.: Geschichtliche Entwicklung der Therapie mit besonderer Berücksichtigung der Naturheilmethoden. In: Krause-Garré: Therapie Innerer Krankheiten Bd. I, pp. 776–815, Jena 1926. — EGLI, M.: Psychosomatik bei den deutschen Klinikern des 19. Jahrhunderts. Zurich 1964. — EREZ, R.: Marshall Hall 1797 bis 1857. Zurich 1963.

163

FIELD, M. J.: Religion and Medicine of the Ga People. Oxford 1937. — FISCHER-HOMBERGER, E.: Hypochondrie. Bern 1970. — FISCHER, Hermann: Mittelalterliche Pflanzenkunde. Munich 1929. — FRANKLIN, A.: Les Médicaments. Paris 1891.

GERHARD, E.: Beiträge zur Geschichte einiger Solaneen. Colmar 1930. — GILG, E., and SCHÜRHOFF, P.: Aus dem Reich der Drogen. Dresden 1926. — GRASSET, H.: La médicine naturiste à travers les siècles. Paris 1911. — GUBSER, A. W.: Charles Barbeyrac und Thomas Sydenham. Zurich 1964.

HAAS, H.: Spiegel der Arznei. Berlin 1956. — HAESER, H.: Lehrbuch der Geschichte der Medizin. 3 vol., Jena 1882. — HAMARNEH, S.: Climax of Chemical Therapy in 10th Century Arab Medicine. Islam 38: 283–288, 1963. — HOLMSTEDT, Bo.: Historical Survey. In Ethnopharmacologic Search for Psychoactive Drugs. Washington 1967, pp. 3–31. — HUMMEL, K.: Herkunft und Geschichte der pflanzlichen Drogen. Stuttgart 1957.

KISSEL, P., and BARRICAUD, D.: Placebos. Paris 1964. — KOELBING, H. M.: Renaissance der Augenheilkunde 1540–1630. Bern 1967. — id.: J. G. Beers "Lehre von den Augenkrankheiten" und die Med. s. Zeit. Clio med 5, 1970. — KREMERS and URDANGS History of Pharmacy revised by G. Sonnedecker, Philadelphia 1963.

LASAGNA, L.: Doctor's Dilemma. New York 1962. — LAUTENSCHLÄGER, C. L.: 50 Jahre Arzneimittelforschung. Stuttgart 1955. — LESKY, E.: Die Wiener Medizinische Schule im 19. Jahrhundert. Graz 1965. — LEWIN, L.: Die Gifte in der Weltgeschichte. Berlin 1920. — LEYDEN, E. v.: Fünfzig Jahre innerer Therapie. Therapeutische Gegenwart 50: 1–10, 1909. — LÖFFLER, W.: Ueber Entwicklungen in der Heilkunde in den letzten 25 Jahren. Festschrift Gesellschaft der Aerzte des Kantons Zürich 1969, pp. 75–128. — LÜTH, P.: Niederlassung und Praxis. Stuttgart 1969 (esp. Chap. 6.2).

MAC-AULIFFE, L.: La thérapeutique Physique d'autrefois. Paris 1904. — MARTINI, P.: Einseitigkeit und Mitte in der Medizin. In: Vom ärztlichen Denken und Handeln. Stuttgart 1956, pp. 58–76.

NEUBURGER, M.: Die Vorgeschichte der antitoxischen Therapie der akuten Infektionskrankheiten. Stuttgart 1901. — id.: Die Lehre von der Heilkraft der Natur. Stuttgart 1926.

PAGEL, W.: Paracelsus. Basle 1958. — PARISH, H. J.: A History of Immunisation. Edinburgh 1965. — PETERSEN, J.: Hauptmomente in der geschichtlichen Entwicklung der Therapie. Copenhagen 1877. — PROKSCH, J. K.: Der Antimerkurialismus. Erlangen 1874.

RAGETH, S.: Die antipyretische Welle. Zurich 1964. — RIVOIR, S.: J. P. Frank als Therapeut. Zurich 1968.

SCHELENZ, H.: Geschichte der Pharmazie. Berlin 1904. — SCHNEIDER, D.: Psychosomatik in der Pariser Klinik von Pinel bis Trousseau. Zurich 1964. — SCHRÖDER, G.: Die pharmazeutisch-chemischen Produkte deutscher Apotheken im Zeitalter der Chemiatrie. Bremen 1957. — SCHRÖDER, W.: Die pharmazeutisch-chemischen Produkte deutscher Apotheken zu Beginn des naturwissenschaftlich-industriellen Zeitalters. Braunschweig 1960. — SIGERIST, H. E.: Studien zur frühmittelalterlichen Rezeptliteratur. Leipzig 1923. — SPAIN, David M.: The complications of modern medical practices. A treatise on iatrogenic diseases. New York 1963. — STAROBINSKI, J.: Histoire du traitement de la mélancolie. Basle 1960. — STICKER, G.: Entwicklungsgeschichte der spezifischen Therapie. Janus 33: 131 ff., 1929. — STRÜMPELL, A.: Zur Charakteristik der gegenwärtigen Therapie. Deutsch. Med. Wochenschrift 48: 1–5, 1922.

TEMKIN, O.: Historical Aspects of Drug Therapy. In: Drugs in Our Society. Ed. by P. Talaley. Baltimore 1964, pp. 3–16.

WALSER, H. H.: A. A. Liébault, Begründer der Ecole de Nancy. Gesnerus 1960, 17: 145–162. — WASSEN, S. H.: Some General Viewpoints in the Study of Native Drugs especially from the West Indies and South America. Ethnos. 1964, pp. 97–120.

ZUMSTEIN, B.: Stoerck und seine therapeutischen Versuche. Zurich 1968.

Appendix

A History of Diet in
Health and Disease

WE WILL actually never know precisely what most people of the past ate. In view of the insufficient data at our disposal a history of diet is therefore rather a history of the rules for nutrition in health and disease than a history of nutrition itself. We subdivide our subject matter into four parts: (1) prehistory, (2) the so-called Greek diet, which lasted into the eighteenth century, (3) the great change in the seventeenth and eighteenth centuries, and (4) the scientific diet of the nineteenth and twentieth centuries.

It is unlikely that many rules for nutrition existed in the early days of mankind. Paleolithic man was probably very hungry most of the time. Constitutionally omnivorous, he probably ate everything that did not kill him. Living on an almost animal level, in view of his very rudimentary technology, he was a so-called collector, i.e., he ate primarily wild plants and small animals, down to insect larvae, snails, etc. How thoroughly he searched his environment for new foodstuffs is illustrated by the fact that in historical times no new edible plants were added to the 700 ones known in prehistory. Paleolithic man discovered during his collecting activities that grains have greater nutritive value than roots, leaves, or fruits and can be stored more easily. He thus invented meals and flours. He had to hunt small animals, as he was rarely a match for the larger ones. To judge from his kitchen refuse, the wild horse seems to have been one of the main objects of his hunting. Prehistoric refuse hills, called Kjökkenmedings in Denmark, instruct us, not without gaps, but objectively concerning nutrition of past times. Wherever possible man consumed fishes and prepared meal from fishes.

He differed from animals in his nutrition in using fire for preparing his food. In general he roasted over the fire or cooked with hot stones in baskets or holes in stones. Pottery was invented only later. When he ate predominantly vegetable food, he salted it.

The most decisive act in the history of nutrition and probably in history in general was the invention of agriculture during the Neolithic. Agriculture was probably invented by grain-collecting women. Later husbandry developed, probably from playing with captured animals. It is surprising that husbandry has by no means everywhere led to milk production. Babylonia, Egypt, and China, although domesticating bovines, have never been milk producers. Husbandry made it possible to inhabit the large steppes. The invention of agriculture and husbandry favored a great increase in population. Our main sources for nutrition and technology in the Neolithic are the objects found below lake dwellings. The first such lake dwellings and objects were discovered in 1851 by Johannes Aeppli in the lake of Zurich. During the Neolithic pottery, metallurgy, and weaving developed. On the basis of these inventions larger and larger cities could develop, first in the Near East.

The first grains to be cultivated were barley and millet. For a long time they were consumed exclusively in the form of a pap. The "Birchermus" is a kind of reminiscence of this nutritional model. But it is also possible to bake pap. This early form of bread still exists in the form of the Scandinavian Knäckebrot, the Jewish matzoh, the Mexican tortilla, and the French crêpes. Eventually fermented bread was invented, in the production of which leaven was used, as in the production of beer. Fermented bread is mentioned in the law of the Babylonian king Hammurabi (2200 B.C.). It is remarkable that the whole rice-consuming Far East has never known bread.

Nutrition, as we have described it, was based on instinct, experience, and taste. Very early other motives became decisive in the choice of foodstuffs: magic, religion, social prestige, and social position. Even today, especially in the lower strata of the population, we find magic considerations in dietary prescriptions. They are based on primitive, mystic ideas—e.g., that the meat of strong animals makes strong, that of weak animals makes weak. These magic ideas served earlier as rationalizations of human cannibalism. Color and form of foodstuffs can equally be interpreted in a magic way: red food gives red cheeks, vegetables resembling genitals increase potency, etc.

Almost all religions have always been closely related to food intake. The religious sacrificial animal is often eaten in a common sacred meal. At the occasion of such a sacred meal, sacred archaic food like millet pap is eaten. It is even possible to eat the god or his sacred animal in the form of baked food. His blood is drunk as wine or another beverage. Man seems to have produced very early fermented beverages, and alcoholic intoxication is often a sacred condition.

Religion plays also a very important negative role in nutrition.

Religious fasting is frequently encountered. The consumption of certain vegetables or animals is forbidden for religious reasons. Such interdictions exist, e.g., in the case of the so-called totem animals, the mystic fathers of the group, or in the case of animals called "unclean." Such religious interdictions are also called taboos. We are most familiar with the Jewish and Mohammedan religious food taboos, and the religious vegetarianism of the Hindu upper class. The question of whether these religious food taboos are rational has been discussed. At first sight the taboo against eating pork makes this impression, but many tribes who eat pork have survived in history. And the Biblical taboo against hares and fishes has no recognizable hygienic foundation. The taboo against pork might just as well reflect the aversion of the nomad to the main source of meat of the agriculturalist. Many of these food taboos are irrelevant from a hygienic point of view, some even detrimental. The existence of such food taboos has brought with it the earliest involuntary dietary experiments. In the Bible it is told that Daniel and his companions refused Babylonian food and lived only on vegetables and water. Their health was good. The Jewish dietary laws are found in the 5th Book of Moses, Chapter 14.

A third irrational element in nutrition is prestige. It is for reasons of prestige that the average Roman ate only white bread, while the wholesome barley was given only to gladiators and punished soldiers. Kings, e.g., in Egypt, ate only very rare and expensive food, while many monks were obliged to beg for their food. Food, especially the food of those strata of the population who can afford it, is of course submitted to fashion.

The irrational element in food survives as religious tradition or as pure tradition. This tradition is often supposedly based on experience, which it is not, or on "theories" which are rationalizations of habits derived from very different sources. Among the Australian aborigines, e.g., old men receive the best parts of the animal, because they are "unhealthy" for women and children. In Germany horse meat is "disgusting," and the Germans actually still abstain from eating the holy animal of their pagan high god Wotan because thousands of their forefathers, who did not do so at the time of Christianization, have been executed. In neighboring France, which was not Christianized in the same fashion, no such prejudices against horse meat exist. The irrational element in nutrition is so strong that, up to the nineteenth century, so-called scientific nutrition did not profit from the numerous experiences in diet that husbandry had provided during the millennia. Only modern science has done so.

All early dietary laws we know about were of a religious nature. It is the Greeks who made the step from a religious to a secular diet. (The Hindus have an excellent diet for the healthy and the sick. Unfortunately it has so far been impossible to date scientifically the beginnings of these Hindu rules.) The great role the Greeks play in our diet is characterized by the fact that we still use for this notion the Greek word. With the Greeks the word "diet" very often meant not only the regulation of the food intake, but the regulation of the whole daily routine—sleep movement, excretion, passions, exposure to air and water. Diet in the narrower as well as in the more extended sense was extremely important to the old Greek physicians. In the Hippocratic book *The Old Medicine* the evolution of medicine is described as an evolution of diet. Supposedly men found raw food unhealthy and invented our normal diet. As this diet proved to be inadequate for sick people, they invented the diet for the sick. Therewith diet was in the beginning at the center of medicine. Hippocratic diet is based on the doctrine of the four humors (blood, phlegm, black gall, yellow gall) and the four qualities (hot, cold, wet, dry). According to the Hippocratic doctrine, disease is a wrong mixture of the humors. Diet helps nature to bring about the return of health through cleaning of the humors. In the following we will study Greek diet in more detail, as it has been dominant for such a long time, and even today traces of it can be found in official or lay dietary rules. The Greek upper class was extremely health-conscious, and therefore diet-conscious. An additional stimulus for dieting for the Greeks was provided by their intensive activities in the field of sports.

The Hippocratic writings (about 400 B.C) contain a special book on normal diet. The order of foodstuffs discussed reflects to a certain extent their rank in the Greek value scale. The author begins with barley, which is "cool and humid," but also "dry." This classification, according to so-called qualities, is found in every dietary prescription up to the eighteenth century. Barley purges. Such characterizations, whether a substance is purging or not, which are very important to those adhering to humoral pathology, are found in all Greek or Greek-influenced dietary prescriptions. The author praises the barley gruel cake and knows barley gruel with water or wine or honey or milk. Wheat is supposedly stronger and less of a purgative. The author discusses fermented and nonfermented bread. Then he surveys beans, peas, millet, and lentils, which are nourishing, constipating, and produce flatulency. Beef meat is strengthening, constipating, and hard to digest. The meat of other animals is lighter and purges. Birds are drier than quadrupeds. Fishes that live near rocks are lighter; those from swamps or rivers are heavier. Fishes are generally regarded as low-grade food, and this Hippocratic prejudice lived very long. Crustaceans purge. Eggs are strengthening, nourishing, and produce flatulency. Cheese is strengthening, nourishing, heating, and constipating. Milk, as a food for adults, is regarded with suspicion and prescribed only in chronic diseases. Butter seems unknown. Oil served to cover the needs in fat. Water is cold and humid; wine and honey are warm and dry. Honey is hard to digest. A very sad lot are vegetables, which all produce flatulency. Garlic is warm and purging, onions are warm and not purging; both are bad. Lettuce is cool and weakening. Celery is a diuretic; asparagus dry and constipating; pumpkin cold, wet, and purging. Carrots are hot and humid. All basically disturb digestion. The same prejudice is maintained in the case of the fruits of trees, e.g., pears. Apples are even harder to digest. Raw apples constipate, cooked ones purge. Among fruits grapes and green figs are still the best. They are warm, humid, and purging. Almonds and nuts are hot and nourishing.

Strong food should be weakened by cooking, wet food should be dried, dry food should be moistened. The Hippocratic writings differentiate between sweet and fat food.

Bread and meat are in the center of this "ideal" diet. Strong reservations exist against fish, fruit, vegetables, and milk. For the majority of the population this diet was of a purely theoretical nature. Only very rich people could afford it. Only very rich people could afford a doctor too. The majority of the population ate much fruit, vegetables, and fish, because these foods were obtainable most easily. Perhaps this was the real reason why the physicians of the rich despised these materials so much, however they rationalized their prejudices.

In the Hippocratic collection another book deals with diet in acute diseases. Here the main dietary prescription is ptisane, i.e., barley gruel. In this book the number of meals is discussed. Should one take one or two per day? The author comes forth with the Solomonic judgment that one should remain faithful to the number of meals one is accustomed to, as each change, e.g., from gruel cake to bread, is dangerous. As beverages in acute diseases the author recommends hydromel (honey with water), oxymel (vinegar with honey water), and wine. The author does not favor pure water. Diet is to be adopted to season. In winter, diet should be dry and warm. Moderation, i.e., not eating too much, is as important as not eating too little or as bodily exercise. The Hippocratic dietary rules contain undoubtedly many valuable and well-observed data. But they also contain proscriptions, like those against fruit, vegetables, milk, fish, and water, which objectively are not justified and which we call, as we lack a better explanation, prejudices.

The fragments of a cookbook in verse, written by Athenaios in the fourth century B.C., provide us with a great amount of information on the nutrition of the Greek upper class. It becomes obvious that gluttony spread more and more. We also know dietary prescriptions by the successors of Hippocrates, such as Diocles, Chrysippus, Praxagoras, and Erasistratus. They all frequently used thirst and hunger as methods of treatment. The most radical author in this respect was Asklepiades. His successors, the so-called methodists, recommended the metasyncritic diet.

The medical textbook of the Roman patrician Celsus, written at the beginning of our era, i.e., about four hundred years after the Hippocratic writings, contains approximately the same ideas. Celsus too deems diet in health and disease extremely important and recommends moderation. His definition of a meal, which should be composed of salted fish, vegetable and meat, is valid only for wealthy people. Bread has replaced for him the barley cake. He subdivides food according to different criteria—e.g., strong (leguminous plants, bread, meat of mammals, cheese, honey), moderately strong (vegetables, birds, fishes), and weak (vegetables on stalks, fruits, snails, mussels). A second classification is into food that produces good humors (milk, wine, fat meat, liver, raw eggs) and food that produces bad humors (millet, leguminous plants, fish, radish, cabbage). Celsus knows that food that forms good humors is not always good for the stomach. Other classifications are into food that is mild and food that is sharp, or food that produces thick, and food that produces thin phlegm. Celsus is interested in the same, mostly fictitious properties dear to Hippocrates—i.e., the formation of humors, qualities (warming, cooling), influence on digestion (favoring flatulency, purging, constipating, diuretic), and sleep production. This latter property he attributes to opium and lettuce. Celsus has also the same prejudices as his predecessors. Only his attitude toward fruits is more positive. The same holds for Aretaios, who was also a great friend of milk. Interesting therapeutic diet prescriptions of Celsus are salt-free diet in kidney disease, liver in night blindness (already prescribed in Egypt and Mesopotamia), milk in pulmonary tuberculosis and poisoning. The latter idea, which is erroneous, survives up to this day in lay circles. Celsus knew also the nutritive clyster, and very often prescribed fasting.

It seems desirable to report here the dietary prescriptions of the great Greek physician who dominated medicine for 1500 years: Galen of Pergamon (130–201). Galen too discussed food in serial order. He too began with the grains from which bread is prepared. For the Romans of his time wheat was the most important. The Greeks still ate barley. He recommends rice only in diarrhea. Leguminous plants he discusses like Hippocrates. The fruits of trees, among which he also counts melons and cucumbers, are, according to him, hard to digest and produce bad humors and fever. He and his father experienced that themselves. On account of his authority this harmful prejudice was believed in up to the eighteenth century. To him the least objectionable fruits are again grapes and figs. The latter, it is true, produce lice. Baked apple is good in digestive troubles. For all other fruits—peaches, apricots, dates, etc.—he has but negative comments. The same holds for vegetables, of which he finds lettuce to be the least dangerous.

The best meat for him is pork. Therefore pork is eaten by athletes. It most resembles human meat. Beef produces "melancholia." Those who are stupid enough to eat the meat of asses or camels resemble these animals. Dog meat was still recommended by Hippocrates and Diocles. Galen turns it down. He produces the well-known prejudices against fishes. All foods contain one of the four qualities or are a mixture of the qualities. The prototype of the mixture is milk. The best foods are bread, pork, fowls, and sea fishes. In acute diseases Galen prescribes ptisane, in phthisis the milk of women. Cold beverages are dangerous. Garlic, onions, cress, leek, and mustard thin out the humors.

The Romans had their own traditional doctrines of diet. Leguminous vegetables must have been extremely popular with them, as evidenced by such leguminous names as Fabius, Lentulus, Piso, and Cicero. The famous censor Cato had two fixed ideas: one that Carthage should be destroyed, the other that cabbage is the best food and the best remedy. The Romans were great friends of cheese. They brought the art of preparing cheese into Switzerland. The Roman upper class was so gluttonous that lawgivers, concerned with the future of the nation, formulated laws against gluttony since 180 B.C. These favored consumption of vegetables, as vegetables were not under these laws, and a rich Roman wanted to serve as many courses as possible. Eventually even in Rome, Greek dietary prescriptions became dominant.

In the beginning of the Middle Ages the old classic civilization was for a while submerged by the invasion of the barbarians and the appearance of Christianity. Nevertheless reminiscences of it survived in medicine as well as in diet; and diet of the Middle Ages continues to be Greek-influenced, whether we study the Western Middle Ages or the Arab Middle Ages. Diet continues to depend on theories of humors and qualities.

Quite a few of the early Christians were very abstemious as far as food is concerned. Some monastic orders continued this tradition. The famous abbess Hildegard of Bingen, who was relatively moderate, nevertheless wanted to give meat only to sick people. The new religion introduced days when meat was forbidden and yearly fastings. The Arabs, too, had their religious dietary prescriptions and their month of fasting. Medieval diet was partially a return to religious diet. In science dietary prescriptions followed the ancient tradition. Through the Crusades some new materials like sugar and distilled liquors were introduced into western European diet. If changed at all, ancient diet became cruder and fuller of exaggerations.

The best-known hygienic-dietetic book of the Middle Ages is the famous *Regimen Salernitanum,* the rule of Salerno, a didactic poem probably written during the eleventh century for a king. It was named after the famous school of Salerno, and some of its verses continue to live as proverbs. Following Hippocrates and Galen the Salernitan rule recommends moderation and avoidance of change. It appreciates wine, but warns that, when taken together with milk, wine will produce "leprosy." Leprosy was at that time so widespread that probably everything could be made responsible for its appearance. Water is regarded as a bad beverage. Pears, apples, beef, and hares are injurious. The first three prejudices are Hippocratic heirlooms, the last seems derived from the Old Testament. Intestines, except those of the pig, are indigestible. Eel without wine causes leprosy. Pears without wine are poisonous. Fresh eggs are healthy. Milk, especially the milk of goats and asses, is allowed except in fever. Cheese should be taken at the end of the meal, as it is cold and hard to digest. Onions are good for the growth of hair.

That is the "wisdom" of the West. As a representative of the East, we choose the eminent Arab-Jewish physician and philosopher Maimonides, who lived during the twelfth century and whose dietetic writings resemble in many parts those of the great Arab-Persian physician Avicenna (eleventh century). Similarities of Maimonides' diet with that of Aldebrandi (thirteenth century, born in Siena, lived in Troyes) are noticeable. Maimonides is against gluttony. The custom of his time is still not to take more than two meals per day. He recommends as wholesome food: wheat bread, lamb, fowl, i.e., a diet for rich people. Noodles, dumplings, and baked gruel have now become unhealthy. All milk products, except cheese, are detrimental. Milk should be taken according to the prescription of Galen, i.e., mixed with honey and salt, which are supposed to prevent coagulation. Most fishes are noxious. Garlic, onions, cabbage, and radishes are unwholesome (the latter had at least been accepted by Avicenna). All tree fruits are, of course, injurious. A faithful follower of this diet was predestined to become a victim of avitaminosis. The question of whether one should drink with meals was answered differently. Avicenna was against it. Faragola, another dietary authority, said one should drink only with meals.

At the end of the Middle Ages a Venetian nobleman, Cornaro (died in 1566 at the age of 100 years), published a book that acquired a quite unusual popularity. In the introduction Cornaro names as the three great evils of his time gluttony, flattery, and Protestantism. He tells that at 35 he had a bad stomach disease. On the advice of his physician he then started living moderately. He never ate to satiety. Since that time he was healthy and endured stress, like trials or a fall from a horse at 70, without difficulty. Once eating 14 ounces instead of 12 ounces of bread, egg yolk, meat, and soup per day and drinking 16 ounces instead of 14 ounces, he became very sick. He never ate tree fruit or fish and did not drink wine in summer. Cornaro's book, which is useful in many ways, is written entirely in the spirit of the tradition of the ancients. Without doubt this tradition contained many valuable observations, and treatment by diet was still the best treatment available. But there is also no doubt, and we have pointed toward this repeatedly in the preceding, that ancient tradition contained a number of dangerous prejudices and errors. We must therefore admit that the judgment of Elmer V. McCollum, famous for his vitamin discoveries, on Hippocrates and the ancient tradition is not unfair: "It is obvious that Hippocrates knew little about the essentials of nutrition, and propagated some unfounded opinions concerning the quality of foodstuffs."

Criticism of the ancient dietary rules had been voiced occasionally even during the Middle Ages, e.g., by Petrarca. During the sixteenth and seventeenth centuries new elements began to penetrate dietary doctrines. Some of these elements were found simply by way of common sense and actual experience others with the help of the still very rudimentary sciences. The change produced by better attention to real experience becomes particularly visible in the changed attitude toward fruit. The Greek prejudice survived nevertheless up to the middle of the eighteenth century. The Parisian medical faculty condemned in 1670 even the "unhealthy" yeast. J. C. Drummond and Ann Wilbraham, in their classic work *The Englishman's Food* (1939), point toward signs of avitaminosis in the English upper class of the seventeenth century. Unlike the real poor, these poor rich people avoided butter and vegetables if possible. Drummond and Wilbraham mention above all xerophthalmia. They also believed that the predominance of bladder stone during this period is explained by an absence of vitamin A in the diet. Stone was very much discussed at that time and was often attributed to the consumption of cheese.

The young physics and the young chemistry of the seventeenth century produced two trends in medicine: iatrophysics and iatrochemistry. The most famous dietary specialist among the iatrophysicists was Santorio Santorio (1566–1632). Santorio did not obtain lasting results, but he put nutrition research on a solid foundation in introducing the balance into this field. He is with good reason always pictured on his balance, for Santorio weighed himself before and after meals as well as his food and his excrements. He found that of eight pounds intake per day he lost five by so-called insensible perspiration; they had gone into the air. The notion of insensible perspiration became for him the criterion of diet. He was opposed to pork, mushrooms, melons, and berries because they reduce insensible perspiration. His rejection of fruits seems to show that he did not always offer new insights, but sometimes new reasons for old prejudices. He was a great friend of mutton. Onions, garlic, and pheasant were recommendable, too, as they furthered insensible perspiration. Fish and cucumbers were unusable. Santorio failed because he tried to solve an essentially chemical problem too early and with purely physical methods.

Among the iatrochemists or chemiatrists we can discern three varieties: those who do not care for diet or do not mention it; those who recommend the old diet in spite of new theories; and finally those who, on the basis of new theories, recommend a new diet.

The founders of iatrochemistry, Paracelsus and van Helmont, belong to the first category. Drugs meant everything to them, diet nothing. Sylvius, Willis, and Dekker just do not mention diet. For Ettmüller diet is a question of quantity and of good chewing. For chemical reasons he recommends a milk diet in scurvy, phthisis, dysentery, and other diseases.

Ramazzini belongs to the second category, who did not apply their new theories to diet and just repeated the old refusal of fruit or cold water.

The third group begins with Sennert. He accepted iatrochemical theories only partially, but his actual diet is new. He shows no longer the old aversion against vegetables, fruit, milk, fish, and water. The Dutchman Blankaart (1650–1702) believed thickening and acidification of the humors to be the main cause of disease. Consequently he prescribed a new, blood-thinning diet. It consisted essentially of much milk, eggs, chicken broth, veal, rice, pike, perch, tea, and chocolate. Not many recommended the latter two beverages during this period. They as well as coffee were fought very energetically for over a hundred years. Blankaart was attacked violently for his milk diet by traditionalists as well as chemiatrists.

During the eighteenth century the prescribing of a diet in disease continued to become rarer and rarer. One can say that the disappearance of diet was proportional to the disappearance of the Greek tradition. Diet was frequently replaced by polypharmacy, especially by clinicians who were iatrochemists. Paradoxically enough the iatrochemists made, in spite of false theories and unserviceable methods (e.g., they distilled foodstuffs in order to elucidate their composition), some positive contributions in the field of diet. The English iatrochemist G. Cheyne (1671–1743), who suffered himself from obesity, was very well known as a dietary specialist. To him acid and alkaline salts were the essential elements in diet. Out of the earth they entered plants, and via plants they entered animal and man. Too much eating and drinking led to an accumulation of salt in the humors, and this in turn produced a "slackening of the fiber." Cheyne therefore prescribed a diet of 8 ounces of meat, 12 ounces of bread and vegetables, and 16 ounces of beer per day. Drummond thinks this diet insufficient. The portions of Cheyne—one foot and one wing of the chicken, three ribs of the mutton, etc.—can still be regarded as hearty. The art of cooking he felt was pernicious, as it seduced to immoderate habits. One should eat only mature or young things, lettuce, fruit, chicken, hares—the difference of this list from a Greek one is noticeable!—as only these things are well digested. Cheyne produced so-called scales of digestibility. Plant-eating animals are more digestible than meat-eaters. Land animals are more digestible than water animals; the white in animal and plant is more digestible than the red, the tasteless more digestible than the acrid. He also constructed a scale of usefulness, which started with grains. The second rank was held by lettuce, spinach, and cabbage; the third by milk and eggs; the fourth by oil, butter, and cheese; the fifth by young chickens, veal, and sheep; the sixth by older animals; the seventh by venison and pork, which should be forbidden for the weak. The list was closed by fish. This did not eliminate the fact that the major part of the English nation had to live to a large extent on fish. One should avoid meat on every third day. Cheyne found that the poor, living mostly on a vegetable diet, were better off than the rich who consumed great quantities of meat. Water was to him the best beverage. He drank moderately coffee and tea; he fought the evil produced by wine and spirits, and turned down lemon juice.

During the eighteenth century the iatrochemists created a theory of neutralization of foods, which was also spread by others, like Forster, Haller, and Smith. This theory of neutralization helped to rehabilitate fruit and vegetables. It claimed that so-called acid fruits neutralized so-called alkaline, easily putrefying albumen. In reality just the opposite is the case. But the decisive thing was that fruit, so essential for health, now became again an official part of a good diet. That this happened on the basis of a false new theory is of very secondary interest. "Acid" milk neutralized also "alkaline" fever; acid cucumbers neutralized alkaline meat. Acid-producing sugar was regarded by many as a danger for the teeth.

In spite of the general tendency to ignore diet, some of the greatest clinicians of the eighteenth century, like Boerhaave of Leyden, Frederic Hoffmann of Halle, and Cullen of Edinburgh, remained faithful to dietary prescriptions. In spite of the fact that their theories were often iatrochemically or iatrophysically influenced, the diet they prescribed was basically the classic Greek diet. This is true especially for Hoffmann. He was such a fanatic partisan of diet that he allowed making an exception to his rule "run away from doctors and drugs" in the case of physicians who prescribed a diet. He participated in the classic prejudices against fish, vegetables, and fruit. Boerhaave insists much less on these prejudices. Cullen adopted a positive attitude toward vegetables, milk, and fish; although he was no iatrochemist, he too explains metabolic processes by hypothetical acids and alkaline substances.

Having studied the fate of classic and chemiatric diet during the eighteenth century, we still have to describe a third diet in this age, which was based less on undeveloped sciences and rather on common

sense, or actual experience. This diet was dear to all who subscribed
to the slogan: "Back to nature." One of the most prominent representatives of this diet was S. Tissot of Lausanne, who published in
1761 the most widely spread popular treatise on medicine. He
emphasizes that the diet of the peasants (bread, thin milk, vegetables, fruit, rarely meat) has almost nothing in common with the
diet of the rich. In fevers Tissot recommends fasting, the drinking
of much water, soups, and fruit juices. He explicitly turns down the
old prejudices against fruit and vegetables. Another famous reformer, F. A. May, subscribes to the same principles. Unzer, an
Enlightenment physician interested in diet, mocks the old attempts
to prevent the coagulation of milk in the stomach. He too recommends fruit, vegetables, and fish for children, and suggests giving
them more substantial food as early as during the first year of life.

The renowned Johann Peter Frank (1787) believed that the
masses were undernourished. He stated that only poor people were
eating vegetables, garlic, onions, and fruit. He defended potatoes,
against which still numerous prejudices were in circulation. Like
his Swiss colleagues, Tissot and Zimmermann, he turned against the
legend that fruit produces dysentery and strongly recommended its
consumption. But even such an enlightened man still believed fish
to be an aphrodisiac and the cause of leprosy. B. Faust, the author
of a widely read catechism of health (1792), recommends vegetables, fruit, fish, and milk. But he believes that the consumption of
warm bread can be fatal. He emphasizes the necessity of cleanliness
in the kitchen, a very important point of view. Like other representatives of the Enlightenment, he shows a strong aversion against tea,
coffee, liquor, and tobacco. To call the dietary ideas of Linné (1742)
or Zückert (1784) products of common sense would be a misnomer
in spite of the fact that they made the one or the other sensible
suggestion. Linné, e.g., believed that cow's milk causes stupidity,
that the consumption of potatoes produces scabies, and sugar pulmonary tuberculosis. For Zückert bread and water are the only foodstuffs that are always healthy. Most meats, leguminous vegetables,
and dumplings have to be avoided. The well-known eclectic Hufeland gives, in his book *Macrobiotic* (1796), some good advice in
dietary matters. As sugar is bad for the teeth, one should rinse one's
mouth after each meal. One should eat more acid vegetables than
meat, so that "the meat gets neutralized and cool and mild blood is

produced." The Swiss prove, in Hufeland's opinion, that one can grow large and strong on a predominantly vegetable diet. Hufeland too recommends fruit, milk, and vegetables, believes fresh bread to be dangerous, and thinks that fish produces cold fever.

Such great therapeutic dietetic improvements of the eighteenth century as the use of fruit, especially citrus fruit, in the treatment and prevention of the widespread scurvy, or the application of cod liver oil, a fish-born substance, against rickets, were possible only through the elimination of Greek dietary prejudices by critical physicians.

Hospital diets are always very revealing in connection with general diet. Therefore in 1954 I had my student Rabenn examine English hospital diets of the eighteenth century, insofar as they were available. In this connection it must be kept in mind that, at that time, hospital patients were without exception paupers. Rabenn's analysis shows a relatively generous use of meat. Of six diets, two had two days without meat, three had three days without meat, one had no day without meat. Bread, cheese, butter, and milk were given liberally. A comparison of these diets with one of 1687, published by Drummond, which was not bad either, shows that the progress made within one hundred years is amazing. The quantity of meat was now four times as large, and these improvements in hospital diets continued. It was very important that, at the end of the eighteenth century, fruit and vegetables entered hospital diets. Still no fish! In the course of the eighteenth century special diets were developed in these institutions. First, one against fever, where much milk was now added to the traditional pap. Then a so-called dry diet and a diet for the unfortunate people who were treated with high doses of mercury against syphilis. Hospital diets of the eighteenth century were adequate, according to Drummond, while diets in workhouses, schools, etc., were often insufficient, especially diets for older children and adolescents.

Diet was very much neglected in the beginning of the nineteenth century. All that leading "reformers" like Brown, Broussais, and Bouillaud had to offer in the way of a "diet" was hunger. Only Graves "fed fevers." Piorry, an otherwise very enlightened therapist, does not even mention diet! Insofar as diet was used, it stagnated and was on a very low level. An authority like Professor Klose admitted in 1825 that children should receive more nourishment, and that fruit and herbs were indicated in fever. On the other hand, he prescribed strict fasting in insanity or syphilis, or lizards against syphilis and cancer, egg yolk in jaundice, and he limited meat to "phlegmatics and melancholics." Professor Feiler (1821) was even more inadequate. With him fruit still produced dysentery, while sugar was very good for the teeth. The chemist Hünefeld, who published a diet in 1841, had, in spite of extensive chemical knowledge, nothing valuable to contribute. The famous medical cookbook of Wiel (1871) still regarded vegetables as unwholesome, potatoes as the cause of scrofula, and salt as the cause of glandular diseases and scurvy. Professor F. A. Hoffmann believed in 1885 that milk was bad for the stomach and that a salt-free diet in kidney disease was unnecessary. While in Great Britain diet still played a certain role through the works of Parish, Combe, and Pereira, in general the old diet was dead and the new scientific diet was not yet born. This was necessarily a very slow process, which got even slower through the aversion of the clinicians against chemistry. Therefore we can talk of an adequate quantitative scientific diet only after 1870, of an adequate qualitative diet only after 1920.

Between the death of the old and the birth of the new scientific diet a gap formed. This gap was, just as in therapeutics, filled by the sectarians. Graham, Schickeysen, Schweninger, and others each had a new, particular, and exclusive diet to prescribe. Sometimes they were successful, especially when they dealt with people who overfed continuously. The trouble was that they elevated half-truths to the rank of dogmas and that their diet showed again clearly religious traits, although their religion was now named "dietary reform" or "natural life."

The new scientific diet starts with the ingenious discovery of the French chemist Antoine-Laurent Lavoisier that respiration is essentially the intake of oxygen and the output of carbon dioxide. Lavoisier saw that here a kind of combustion takes place, that when oxygen is taken in, the same quantity of heat is produced as in burning coal, and that the quantity of oxygen intake changes according to activity, food, or rest. These discoveries of Lavoisier between 1777 and 1789 made possible a quantitative examination of metabolism. It became possible to classify foodstuffs according to their combustion value in calories.

The second basic element of a new scientific diet was the chemical knowledge of the basic foodstuffs. The English physician and chemist Prout brought in 1827 some clarity into this field in claiming three basic foodstuffs: "albumins, oils, and saccharin" corresponding to our proteins, fats, and carbohydrates. One year before Prout, Parish had still claimed nine basic foodstuffs.

sugar

The sugars became better known through the conversion of starch into grape sugar by the pharmacist Kirchhoff in St. Petersburg in 1812, the discovery of blood sugar by Schmidt in 1844, and through Claude Bernard's work after 1856 on glycogen and sugar metabolism in the body.

The knowledge of fats starts with the discovery of Chevreul in 1814 that fats are composed of different fatty acids and glycerin. (Chevreul, by the way, died in 1889 at the age of 102 years.) Liebig showed later that the body can transform carbohydrates into fat. Fortunately he did not draw any mystical conclusions from this fact, as might have been suggested by the then prevailing notion of organic chemistry. Organic chemistry was regarded at that time as a "vital chemistry," submitted to special laws. The synthesis of urea from nonorganic material by Wöhler in 1828 put an end to these notions. After Wöhler, organic chemistry has been only the chemistry of C-molecules.

Albuminous materials had been seen as a unit by the Dutchman Mulder. After 1842 the famous German chemist J. Liebig became particularly interested in proteins. Originally he thought, like Mulder, that there existed only one protein. Liebig (1803–1873) studied all three foodstuffs, but his favorite studies were on proteins. He demonstrated that the decomposition of protein in the body could be determined by the N-values in urine. In 1816 the French physiologist Magendie had fed dogs with pure carbohydrates or fats and experimentally shown that N-containing foodstuffs are absolutely necessary for survival. Liebig called protein a "plastic foodstuff," because he assumed that it was used up by the functioning muscles. Fick and Wislicenus showed in their ascent of the Faulhorn in 1866 that increased labor is not accompanied by increased decomposition of protein in the body. Liebig called the other foodstuffs "respiratory substances," i.e., in his opinion they produced heat. The overemphasis on proteins in the diet of the second half of the nineteenth century is undoubtedly a consequence of the erroneous concepts of Liebig.

A lively discussion concerning the minimum requirements for protein arose between Liebig's most eminent pupil, Voit (1831–1908), and young critics like Chittenden. Around 1880 Voit formulated the necessary minimum as 118 grams protein, 56 grams fat, and 500 grams carbohydrates. Better understanding of protein problems developed when the composition of proteins by peptones and the composition of peptones by amino acids were discovered. In 1872, O. Nasse showed that tyrosine is an essential amino acid without which the body cannot exist.

Metabolism research was continued after Lavoisier, but encountered great technical difficulties. The notion of metabolism is formulated as "Stoffwechsel" by Gmelin and Tiedemann in their famous book of 1836. Boussingault established in 1839 the first balance sheet in calories. Reignault and Reiset determined the respiratory quotient. All this was done with animals. Voit and Pettenkofer were eventually able to study these phenomena in man with their improved apparatus between 1866 and 1879. These studies were continued by the disciples of Voit, especially Rubner, who established isodynamic values of foodstuffs.

Necessary for the formulation of a new diet was, of course, a better knowledge of digestion. Up to the nineteenth century digestion was regarded either as a purely mechanical process or a process of putrefaction. These errors began to be eliminated after the experiments of Réaumur and Spallanzani at the end of the eighteenth century. They showed that digestion was a chemical process. An important stage in the further understanding of digestion was the observations of Beaumont in 1833 in a case of fistula of the stomach. They led directly to the work of Pavloff. Of fundamental importance was the discovery of the different enzymes of digestion, such as pepsin (Schwann) and trypsin (Danilevski).

How did diet look at the end of the nineteenth century, when it tried to use these scientific discoveries? Diet had undoubtedly again gained more importance, all the more as the amazing discoveries of the bacteriologists had so far not borne therapeutic fruits. The new diet was based on caloric calculations and was quantitatively rather reliable. Special diets were developed for different professions, ages (especially infants), and sexes. The development of special diets in special diseases had increased tremendously since the eighteenth century. The most important diet of this kind was still the fever diet. In

1908, in the diet textbook of Strauss, it was the last recommended in the list of special diets. Fever diet was at the time of the antipyretic wave a strictly liquid diet. In all other respects it was meager, too. The dietary alcoholism, which had spread everywhere from England, fortunately started disappearing around the turn of the century. Another important diet was the one for convalescents. It was extremely rich in proteins, but fruit was much neglected. There was a difference between the so-called régime blanc and régime rouge. Milk diets were very popular. Milk, not so long ago something of little value, became now a kind of dietary panacea. The bland kidney diet, too, contained much milk. An important diet was the gastrointestinal diet, consisting mainly of rice soup, farinaceous food, milk, which was also given as clysters, and eggs. There were still dietitians, like Wiel, who turned down potatoes as a "food for proletarians." The reducing diets were of great practical importance, as the upper classes lived in a state of chronic overfeeding. The reducing system of the layman Banting (1863) became very popular with physicians. The opposite of the reducing diet was the fattening diet. The fattening diet was a widespread attempt to stem the most frequent disease of the time, pulmonary tuberculosis. Following the work of an American, Silas Weir Mitchell (1870), the fattening diet was also used against the most frequent functional disease of the time, neurosis.

The diet for diabetics consisted, as far back as Rollo (died 1809), predominantly of meat. As the role of carbohydrates in diabetes became better known, milk and farinaceous food were forbidden. Gout diets were based on meat or milk. Cardiac diets attempted above all reduction of liquid intake. In this field the Karrel cure became very fashionable for a while. Sodium chloride intake was limited too. There existed furthermore pulmonary, nervous, cancer (vegetarian!), and liver diets.

In 1881 a young Russian named Lunin, working in the laboratory of Gustav von Bunge in Basle, tried to raise young rats with a diet composed of the "essential" foodstuffs. The experiment failed. The rats died. Ten years later similar experiments of another Bunge disciple, Socin in Basle, had the same results. But neither the students nor their teacher concluded from these experiments that the so-called complete diet was not complete. This insight grew only out of the work of Eijkman (1889), Pekelharing (1905), Hopkins (1906), and Stepp (1909), who found that natural food contains minimal quantities of so far unknown essential substances. These substances were baptized vitamins by Casimir Funk. After 1912 vitamins A, B, C, D, etc., were discovered by McCollum, Steenbock, Osborne, Mendel, Windaus, and others. In these years also realized was the vital importance of inorganic elements in very small quantities, of essential amino acids, etc. On these foundations eventually a complete scientific diet became possible. While in 1900 only five basic elements had been known, in 1950 their number had risen to forty. The discoveries of molecular pathology also influenced strongly certain diets. In idiopathic galactemia, e.g., it has become possible to protect the child against numerous pathological developments, included dementia, by simple omission of milk sugar from the diet.

The experiences of the first World War brought about certain changes in the chronic overfeeding of the upper classes. During that war it became quite clear that sometimes it is healthier to eat less. Another factor unfavorable to overfeeding was the new fashion of bodily appearance, which had to be "sportsmanlike" in men and women. While after the first World War the upper classes ate less, the lower classes ate more. In the so-called capitalist countries a certain leveling off of the differences in diet with a tendency toward a "classless" nutrition has developed. Class differences in the field of nutrition are much less pronounced than those in the field of living quarters. Class differences in diet, which still exist outside of the so-called Western world, have existed since the beginnings of humanity and have sometimes been quite extraordinary. As we have seen, from a dietary point of view often two "nations" were living in the same country. It is typical in this respect that during the scurvy epidemics of the eighteenth century on board ship officers, whose food was different from that of the men, remained healthy most of the time. During the first World War a saying circulated in the German army which alludes to this class difference in diet: "Gleicher Lohn und gleiches Essen, wär der Krieg schon lang vergessen." (If we all had the same pay and the same food, the war would long be over.) As this situation is not so far removed in time, prestige elements in the choice of food and beverages still play a great role today.

Bibliography

ACKERKNECHT, E. H.: History of metabolism. Ciba Symposia 6: 1814–1844, Summit, N.J. 1944. — CARL, El.: Die Diätbehandlung Kranker im 19. Jahrhundert. Diss. Düsseldorf 1938. — CARSON, G.: Cornflake Crusade. New York 1957. — DEUTSCH, R. M.: The Nuts among the Berries. New York 1961. — DRUMMOND, J. C., and WILBRAM, A.: The Englishman's Food. London 1964. — DUSTMAN, M.: Die Geschichte der Ernährungstherapie im Altertum. Diss. Düsseldorf 1938. — EDELSTEIN, L.: The Dietetics of Antiquity, in: Ancient Medicine, Baltimore 1967. — GOTTSCHALK, A.: Histoire de l'Alimentation et de la Gastronomie, 2 vol. Paris 1948. — HINTZE, K.: Geographie und Geschichte der Ernährung. Leipzig 1934. — LICHTENFELT, H.: Die Geschichte der Ernährung. Berlin 1913. — LUSK, Graham: Nutrition. New York 1964. — MAURIZIO, A.: Histoire de l'alimentation végétale. Paris 1932. — McCOLLUM, E. V.: A History of Nutrition. Boston 1937. — PETERSON, J.: Zur Geschichte der Ernährungstherapie, in: LEYDEN, E. v.: Handbuch der Ernährungstherapie. Leipzig 1903. — RABENN, W. B.: Hospital diets in 18th century England. J. Am. Diet. Assoc. 30, 1954, 1216–1221. — ROTHSCHUH, K. E.: Krankenkost in alten Tagen. Deutsch. Med. Journ. 12, 117–123, 1961. — SCHOLLE, K.: Gesundheitsführung bei Linné. Diss. Bonn 1962. — TEMKIN, O.: Nutrition from classical antiquity to the baroque. Human Nutrition Monograph III. New York 1962, pp. 78–96.

Index